Patrick Kingsley, MBBS, MRCS, LRCP, FAAEM, DA, DObst, RCOG, helped establish the clinical pharmacology department at Fisons Pharmaceuticals in 1970, where he was responsible for international research, particularly involving asthma. Trained at St Bartholomew's Hospital and experienced in many aspects of orthodox medicine, he is also a founder member of the two professional bodies for nutritional and environmental medicine. He is Chief Medical Officer of *Foresight*, the association for the promotion of preconceptual care.

Principal author of the chapter on the asthma drug Intal (sodium cromoglycate) in the medical textbook *Allergy, Principles and Practice*, he has also written several popular books on food intolerance and illness, including the treatment of cystitis.

Dr Kingsley is married with two sons and has a private practice in Leicestershire.

Ian Stoakes trained as a teacher in the 1970s, concentrating on behaviourally disturbed children. After running a unit for mentally handicapped children he was employed by the Home Office as principal of a secure unit.

During the 1980s he worked for a number of charities, primarily involved with children and nutrition. These twin interests were exploited during his time as Chief Executive of the Dietary Research Foundation, which conducted a multi-national trial investigating the relationship between nutrition and intelligence.

Ian Stoakes is married with two young sons and lives in Shere, Surrey.

THE NUTRON DIET

PATRICK KINGSLEY AND
IAN STOAKES

PENGUIN BOOKS

PENGUIN BOOKS

Published by the Penguin Group
Penguin Books Ltd, 27 Wrights Lane, London W8 5TZ, England
Penguin Books USA Inc., 375 Hudson Street, New York, New York 10014, USA
Penguin Books Australia Ltd, Ringwood, Victoria, Australia
Penguin Books Canada Ltd, 10 Alcorn Avenue, Toronto, Ontario, Canada M4V 3B2
Penguin Books (NZ) Ltd, 182–190 Wairau Road, Auckland 10, New Zealand

Penguin Books Ltd, Registered Offices: Harmondsworth, Middlesex, England

First published privately 1994
Published in Penguin Books 1994
1 3 5 7 9 10 8 6 4 2

NuTron is a registered trade mark owned by Nutron Ltd. It is used under licence in the
United Kingdom by The Individual Diet Company Ltd, and Food Tolerance Testing Ltd,
The Old Mill, The Street, Albury, Guildford, Surrey GU5 9AZ. Tel: 0483 203555.
Fax: 0483 203456. The NuTron Test is the subject of patent applications worldwide.

Printed in England by Clays Ltd, St Ives plc

Contents

FOREWORD
Losing a battle...winning a war
by Nina Myskow

It was a lifetime's obsession. I fought - and lost - the battle with my weight until I was over forty. Then one day, sitting on a beach in the Caribbean, I decided I'd finally had enough. At five feet two-and-a-half inches and twelve-and-a-half stone there's only so much you can overcome with personality. I realised that the life I longed to lead was rapidly passing me by. I was determined to change, to become the person I felt on the inside. And I did. Through sheer bloody hard work, sensible eating and daily exercise, I managed to lose three stone.

I'm proud of that. And even happier that for the last five years I've more or less kept it off - if not without a constant struggle. Through years of trying every new fad diet I know the calorie, fat and fibre content of every food and drink. But I enjoy life - and pink champagne - too much to be sensible all the time. I'd relax, let things go slightly, and suddenly half a stone would appear from nowhere. Then I'd be back to existing on tedious salads and cottage cheese and stepping up my exercise regime. Dieting alone never works for me because I have the metabolism of a slug - it needs to be prodded with the big stick of exercise. Fortunately, I really enjoy my daily aerobics and conditioning classes. You may end up sweaty and exhausted, but you do feel smug and virtuous.

In the summer of 1993 I was up to ten-and-a-half stone, feeling depressed and about to grit my teeth and

1

start all over again when Sally Ann Voak, Slimming Editor of 'The Sun', asked me to be a guinea-pig in what I was told was a revolutionary approach to losing weight. While I was willing to try anything, I wanted to know what was involved - which is how I came to meet Ian Stoakes, of The Individual Diet Company, which developed The NuTron Diet.

What he had to say was intriguing. All of us, virtually without exception, are intolerant to some foods - and it's different foods for different people. Because we're not aware of these intolerances we go on eating the things we shouldn't, which has an adverse effect on our body chemistry. And this causes weight gain, most of it in the form of retained fluid. Why this happens - and why some people aren't prone to internal leaking - isn't understood. But enlightened doctors, who've treated certain medical conditions such as arthritis and multiple sclerosis by changes in diet, have been aware of it for decades. And they were aware of something else: eliminating the foods to which their patients were intolerant not only brought pronounced improvement in health but was invariably accompanied by significant weight losses.

Then why hadn't someone already based a commercial diet on food intolerances for ordinary dieters? Because no-one had found an easy, sure-fire way of identifying food intolerances. That, however, was exactly what The Individual Diet Company had done - by originating a method of analysing any individual's blood sample against a range of common foods. There was another piece of information which I thought was startling: once you'd removed from your diet the foods to which you were intolerant, you could eat as much as you liked of the other tested foods and you'd still lose weight.

The more I listened, the more convinced I became that everything Ian said made sense.

I was fascinated when I saw the results of my blood test and the list of foods that I was intolerant to: tannin (tea, red wine, prunes, currants, raisins, plums), baker's and brewer's yeast, coffee, corn, mushrooms, cheese, peanuts, curry powder, sesame seeds, milk and - wait for it - lettuce and cucumber. Lettuce and cucumber had been making me fat? All those salads I'd been forcing down had been doing me no good at all! If The NuTron Diet worked for me, however, I'd never have to come face to face with another lettuce leaf...

I was thrilled *not* to be intolerant to white grapes - white wine and champagne weren't off limits.

I lost five pounds in the first week without trying. I did get coffee withdrawal symptoms - working at home I'd been used to drinking it all day long - which gave me a thumping headache for four days, something I never have. I just pretended it was one hell of a hangover. After that it was straightforward. By the time I went on holiday five weeks later I'd dropped twelve pounds and could hardly believe it. To achieve that kind of loss in the past I'd practically had to starve myself and exercise non-stop.

Holidays are for relaxing but, because of my weight problems, I've never been able to let myself go like other people without disastrous results. This year, my partner Grant and I went to St Lucia in the West Indies (where my change of heart had begun to change my life all those years before). It was one of those all-inclusive holidays where you lie on the beach all day and just put up a flag every time you want a drink.

We fell head first into Piña Coladas. They taste like scrummy milk shakes, but they're a lethal mix of rum, coconut cream and pineapple juice. In the bad old days

I'd never have dared risk them. Rum is made from sugar, which years of dieting told me to avoid. As for coconut cream, I'd have said it was so fattening you'd put on pounds just smelling it. Still, neither was on my banned list so I thought: go for it. We did, too, six or more each a day. We practically smeared Piña Colada all over our bodies! And I ate - the food was wonderful. I stuck rigidly to my list, but that gave me a lot of leeway. I can still taste the Caribbean roast pork from the barbecue night - and the crackling which I'd never, ever have allowed myself before...

I steeled myself for the worst when we got back home. By rights I should have been at least half a stone in disgrace. But the scales showed I hadn't put on an ounce.

Believe me, I've tested my diet to the limit and I know it works, as long as I avoid the things I'm not supposed to have. You pay the price instantly if you ignore that rule or just don't use your head. Ten days into my diet we went out for a Chinese meal and next morning I'd gained four pounds. I could have wept. What I hadn't realised was that the dishes were cooked in peanut oil and sesame oil - a couple of the 'trivial' things on my list. Still, Sally Ann Voak had a worse experience. She went on a weekend trip to France, deliberately ate some of her banned foods to see what would happen - and put on six pounds! And she's a slim, healthy woman who's never had a real weight problem.

Obviously, I've written from my own experience, but in the course of my involvement with The Individual Diet Company I've met dozens of people who've achieved results every bit as good as mine, and better. One chap lost five stone in two months while eating three slap-up meals a day. Another had only lost nine pounds (in less than a week, mind!) when I spoke to him, but he was over the moon - before he'd been tested for his food intolerances he'd been on a 500-calorie diet which consisted of little more than fat-free yoghurt, he'd been swimming a mile every morning and every evening - and still he'd put on weight.

As someone who's suffered for over thirty years, I know the misery being overweight can cause. Being overweight is a major problem in this country. Britain's Chief Medical Officer has warned that the sharp rise in the number of people seriously overweight was undermining a drive to improve the nation's health. You can't argue with the statistics: in 1991, 13% of men aged sixteen to sixty-four were obese (that is 20% over their ideal weight) against 7% four years earlier; and 15% of women, against 13% across the same period. In the autumn of 1993, an American study published in the 'New England Journal of Medicine' showed that obese young men are 11% less likely to get married - a figure which rises to 50% among obese young women.

Being overweight can be utter misery. Whatever brave face you put on it - and I was Jolly Old Nina for years - inside it's a very different story. What's awful about being overweight is that is causes such despair - trying to do up a zip that won't meet, or suddenly catching sight of yourself in a shop window. There's such guilt when the pounds go on. And such self-disgust when they won't come off. And such a loss of self-esteem and confidence.

But I believe it no longer has to be like that. Because The NuTron Diet is the breakthrough that changes the business of slimming from the hit-and-miss affair it's always been - and perhaps for the first time in your life puts you in control of your body. Already I know of three hospitals, a number of consultants in private practice and over a hundred GPs who are using the blood test in association with weight loss and other conditions. So are health and fitness clubs all over the country.

The Individual Diet Company is gearing up so as to be able to deal with two thousand samples a day by the end of 1994.

The NuTron Diet is of huge importance in the treatment of various medical conditions, one of which is pre-menstrual tension. Before I started the diet, I was told it would almost certainly alleviate my PMT symptoms. Frankly, I didn't believe that. I've always suffered from PMT. Once a month my life was a misery. I was physically clumsy, I'd get mentally confused, unable to remember names and words - and in floods of tears at the slightest thing. I was never outwardly aggressive - I turned it all against myself. For five days I'd live in a fog of self-doubt and depression. And physically I felt so bloated I thought I'd explode like a volcano.

All that went - instantaneously. And hasn't returned. I feel like a normal human being all month. Not only haven't I suffered PMT since taking up The NuTron Diet, nor has Grant!

Altogether, what The NuTron Diet has done for me is almost beyond words and I've become a bit of an evangelist on the subject - I know from those who've written to me at 'The Sun', or who've responded when I've talked about the diet on TV and radio, just how desperate many people are for help.

It's now six months since I took my own test. I've shed a stone and people keep telling me, "gosh you look good," or "I can't believe how much weight you've lost," or (so help me) you look younger." Having accepted for so long that life was unfair - and that I was just one of those unfortunates who had to eat less than others - I have to say I think justice has been done at last.

The NuTron Diet has changed my life. It can change yours, too.

ALL OTHER DIETS ARE OBSOLETE!

We could build our case gradually, present the evidence, come to our conclusions. You, however, want to know what we're saying now, and in words of one syllable.

So let us tell you:

- **Food intolerance exists**
- **Probably everyone without exception has it**
- **It is a major cause of excess weight**
- **Different people are intolerant to different foods**
- **A test has been developed that simply and accurately identifies the foods to which YOU individually are intolerant**
- **The test also tells you which foods you can safely eat - the foods to which you are NOT intolerant**
- **It is probable that eliminating your intolerant foods and eating from your safe foods is all that you have to do to be slim**

Does it sound too good to be true? Well, there's more. If the weight you need to shed is in stones rather than in pounds this "double whammy" test will see to it that the excess simply drops off. And that the hard-core fat, which is the hardest to shift -

and those unsightly areas of cellulite - will go, if less dramatically, *and won't come back.*

* * *

The vast majority of dieters are women. Nine out of ten women try to lose weight at some time in their life. Half the women everybody knows are probably on a diet right at this minute. Some women are dieting permanently. More men than women (40% against 32%) are overweight but for reasons beyond the scope of this book fewer of them care to diet - though in recent years their number has increased.

It's to be applauded that so many people strive to lose weight - excess poundage on members of either sex is not only unattractive it's medically unsound (a recently published Office of Health Economics paper likened being ten pounds overweight to smoking twenty cigarettes a day in terms of the risk to your health). What is a matter of regret is that for so long the dietary methods which have been available have so frequently let people down.

Over many years, diets have been brutal in their disappointment, falling short of what they say they will deliver. Excess weight is not removed without a major struggle; perhaps more cruelly, even when it is, it creeps back; either way leaving the dieter angry, frustrated - and guilty for having failed, which, indeed, can then become part of the problem. Promises implied, promises broken - after the expenditure of time, effort, inconvenience and money. How many women fail at every diet they try and go on to the next and the next with the same result? More than a quarter of people attending slimming clubs find that they have to return time and again. And what about those too disappointed to come back? And those too ashamed to have gone in the first place?

There are all kinds of diets, high fibre, low salt or fat, milk or fruit, nutritional drink diets, diets that pair types of food, diets that involve eating certain foods only at specific times of day or year, diets that put you on high energy pills and fat-busting pills. And many more, including those which involve exercise. Most of these are put forward in good faith, some are based on questionable science, a few are nonsensical - rapid loss diets which subject an average woman, who needs 2,000-2,500 calories a day, to a quarter of her requirement or even less, are simply unsustainable at best and hazardous at worst.

When it comes down to it, however, virtually all diets have this in common: they limit your intake of calories. Weight gain, so the theory goes, is caused by calories which are not converted into energy - which, to put it another way, you don't use up by living - and which are turned into fat instead. Do without the calories you don't need for living, so the theory goes, and you'll lose weight.

The theory has dominated our eating habits for over half a century, ever since two American doctors, Newburgh and Johnston at the University of Michigan, proclaimed that "obesity stems not from a deficient metabolism but from a diet too rich in calories."

Simply put, this means that if your body needs 2,500 calories a day to keep it in running order and you feed it 2,000, it will find the extra 500 by making a "withdrawal" from its fat reserves - with consequent weight loss. Obversely, if you feed your body 3,000 calories, it will deposit as fat the 500 it doesn't require.

What's wrong with this argument is that it makes no allowances for the fact that the body adjusts to its circumstances. Of course, someone needing 2,500 calories will initially experience weight loss on 2,000 calories. But then the body not only gets accustomed to its lessened supply and lives within its means, it takes the precaution of not using up all of what it's now getting. *It puts a bit aside as a precaution - as stored fat. You eat less...and yet you gain weight.*

"Burning off" calories through exercise is just as fallacious. All that exercise does is use up the short-term fuel (glycogen) which you get from your consumption of carbohydrates - it doesn't touch the fat stored for long-term use. And your body adjusts to regular exercise in exactly the same way as it adjusts to reduced calorie intake - it gets used to it and simply provides more short-term fuel to meet the demand. True, that means less long-term fat goes into store - but some still does and what's already there stays where it is. You can gain weight while exercising just as you can while reducing your calories.

In his best-selling book 'Dine Out and Lose Weight', Michel Montignac describes the theory of calorie counting as "probably the greatest scientific swindle of the 20th century." And he has our whole-hearted support. Not only is calorie counting as a means of weight loss dangerously simplistic, it has no validated scientific basis whatsoever - we've researched the medical literature without turning up any validated test. It is quite significant that all calorie-controlled dietary methods are currently being investigated in the USA by the Food and Drug Administration for making unsubstantiated claims.

What *we* are saying - and it's not an unsubstantiated claim - is that food intolerance is the enemy within, not the calories. Certainly, excess calories can cause excess weight. But reducing them is an answer to the wrong problem. The problem that needs to be addressed is: Why has your body lost control of the way it should regulate the calories?

The answer is that food intolerance has knocked the body's mechanisms out of balance. Once the intolerance has been taken care of, the mechanisms will normalise and, automatically, you will stop craving carbohydrates. Without any effort of will, you will consume fewer of them. At the same time, more energy will build up in you and your body will expend that energy because you become more active. You can forget the calories - you've handed the job back to your body. *And you will lose weight - and prevent its return - while eating as much as your appetite dictates.*

* * *

It's time we explained exactly how your body reacts when you eat a food to which you are intolerant.

Before food can be absorbed by the blood and used to nourish the cells of the body, it has to be converted in the digestive system, or alimentary canal, which begins at the mouth and goes right through the trunk. Digestion starts in the mouth and continues in the stomach and small intestine - where absorption mainly takes place.

Carbohydrates consist of sugar or starch and starch has to be turned into sugar before the body can use it. This process is begun by an enzyme, ptyalin, which is in the saliva. Once in the stomach, the food is mixed with gastric juice, poured from millions of tiny glands that contain hydrochloric acid and several enzymes, the most important of which, pepsin, helps to digest proteins such as eggs and lean meat. A little water, some fruit sugars and alcohol are absorbed in the stomach, but the majority moves on into the duodenum to continue the process of digestion.

The time the stomach takes to digest a meal varies from perhaps one hour to five. Once it's digested, the food, now in a liquid state and referred to as chyme, passes into the small intestine. Here, bile from the liver acts on the fats in the chyme and juices from the pancreas - which also produces the hormone, insulin - do the major work of breaking down all the ingredients. There are small glands in the lining of the small intestine that contribute other digestive juices.

The area of the small intestine is very much increased because it's lined with tiny, finger-shaped objects called villi that contain both capillaries - the tiniest blood vessels - and other vessels filled with lymph fluid. The lymphatic vessels absorb fat; the capillaries take nourishment from the chyme and pass it into the bloodstream.

Food that has not been absorbed now lies in the large intestine before passing from the body as waste. It is during this period that water is absorbed and carried by the bloodstream to the kidneys.

Any food to which you're intolerant interferes with this process, making something happen that shouldn't: your intestinal wall becomes porous.

Embedded in the tissues throughout the body are cells that are shaped rather like a Walt Disney beehive and which, rather quaintly, are named mast cells after a bag in which Americans collect mast - or beech - nuts. These are especially common in the tubes leading to the lungs, in the nose and in the gut.

The mucous membrane of the gut wall contains millions of mast cells. When these are aggravated by the food - or foods - to which they are intolerant they pop open, releasing chemicals that cause the gut wall to become permeable. Particles of incompletely digested food substances, including fat globules, cross over directly into the bloodstream. Once there, they attack the white blood cells, concentrating on the neutrophils.

Apart from the liquid in the blood, there are three groups of cells: the red blood cells that carry the oxygen around the body, the platelets that are primarily responsible for clotting when you cut or injure yourself, and the white blood cells that look after defence mechanisms. The white blood cell group comprises five different cell types, three of which have a granular appearance and are therefore called granulocytes: eosinophils, basophils and neutrophils. These are responsible for defending the body against invaders - viruses and bacteria - which they attack, engulf and destroy. The monocytes and lymphocytes, which aren't granular, sweep up the debris that results from these skirmishes.

Viruses and bacteria come from outside the body and the neutrophils, which make up by far the largest number of the white cells and are the first into any fight, know what to do against them. But this "invasion" of food particles is an inside job and, faced with it, the neutrophils become confused. Instead of attacking, they allow themselves to be attacked. And the chemical granules that they contain - which are extremely toxic - fall out like marbles.

This little Star Wars is hardly life threatening. Under attack the neutrophils expand, shrink, swim around injured, explode, but their life term is only ten hours anyway - the body is reproducing eighty million neutrophils *an hour*. If your body didn't produce new cells your system would gradually break down. But that doesn't happen. Your body goes on manufacturing millions of new cells and puts them into service. And while you're not eating - or fortuitously avoid the foods that make you intolerant when you do eat - the neutrophils go their way, healthily and usefully. And the body takes advantage of the opportunity to repair earlier damage, the filter systems, the kidneys and the liver, doing their best to clean up the mess, the one taking out water-soluble waste, the other converting fat-soluble waste chemicals into water-soluble ones for excretion through the kidneys. Whenever you eat whatever it is that sets up a reaction, however, the whole insidious cycle begins again.

The difference between the mast cells and the neutrophils is that where the former are anchored in place, the latter are circulating in the blood. As the neutrophils are degranulated by the "invasion" of food particles, their "marbles" pollute the bloodstream - giving you, in effect, a minor case of blood poisoning.

An unholy trinity of consequences can be conjured up by food intolerance: fluid, candida and hypoglycaemia.

Of them, **fluid** is probably the slimmer's biggest enemy. Fluid is heavy - a pint of water weighs a pound and a quarter. Anyone drinking ten cups of tea or coffee a day in half-pint mugs is taking in six and a quarter pounds in weight. Fluid is also an ingredient of solid foods and, very obviously, goes into such things as gravy and custard. The majority of all this is passed out in the normal way. But in many people, particularly the very overweight, a proportion isn't - because the toxic "marbles" spilled from the neutrophils into their bloodstream are causing something else to happen: they're making the capillaries at the periphery of the arterial system all over the body, leak in exactly the same way as the gut wall has leaked. Fluid is being pushed out into the body tissues instead of being returned to the kidneys. And there's no easy way of getting that fluid back to where it should go.

MOST OVERWEIGHT PEOPLE AREN'T FAT, THEY'RE WATERLOGGED.

Some people's bodies are leakier than others. Some people are intolerant to one food that will make them leak copiously where someone else may be intolerant to twenty foods and hardly leak at all - leakage depends on your pre-disposition and you can do no more about it than you can about your height or the natural colour of your hair. Some other people who are food intolerant won't experience leaky capillaries at all - and they may not be overweight - but they're likely to pay a price in other ways. The toxins circulating in their blood may prise open the mast cells in the lungs, for instance, leading to the onset of asthma. The fact is, food intolerance has been implicated in a wide variety of chronic conditions including not only asthma but arthritis, irritable bowel syndrome and cystitis, and in a range of childhood conditions such as colic, glue ear and tonsillitis. Eradicating food intolerance can alleviate or totally remove these disorders. Anyone suffering both a chronic condition *and* overweight is likely to find the outcome of removing their intolerance little short of miraculous.

How much overweight is due to fluid accumulation? If you're the sort of person who feels bloated after a meal or whose weight shoots up after coming off a diet then fluid accumulation is quite certainly your problem, as it is for any woman who experiences a gain of more than a pound or two during her pre-menstrual phase.

Some excess weight, of course, *is* fat. As every battle-hardened dieter knows, fat, which takes a long time to be deposited, is hard to shift and most people have scant success. That is especially the case where cellulite is concerned.

Cellulite is a form of fluid accumulation - fluid that's been leaked by the capillaries and become trapped in areas of cells almost always centred on the buttocks, thighs, or upper arms. The superficial tissues of the body are attached to the deeper tissues by fibrous strands. The knobbly, puckered texture that embarrasses so many women is caused by the area in between these becoming unreasonably stretched by fat and fluid that shouldn't be there. Imagine a wire-mesh hanging flower basket in which the soil represents the deeper tissue, the sheet of black plastic that holds in the soil represents the superficial layers - and the bumps where the soil pushes the plastic through the wire mesh (something that can become exaggerated when the basket receives a good watering) is the cellulite, and you have a pretty good idea of what occurs. Women suffer from cellulite, men seldom do. Women have twice the amount of fatty tissue as men, but that isn't the reason: cellulite results from the action of the female hormone oestrogen, particularly at puberty, during pregnancy and at the menopause. Even young women who are not fat can and do have cellulite.

And every woman who has, is a victim of food intolerance.

The second of the slimmer's enemies is **candida.**

Candida albicans is a yeast, a single-celled micro-organism that exists naturally on the skin and mucous membranes of human beings and which is one of the many micro-organisms, sometimes called the flora, which colonise the gastro-intestinal tract. The vast majority of these bacteria have benefits, preventing other, unfriendly kinds - like candida - from gaining a potentially damaging foothold, as well as providing us with some vitamins and aiding digestion.

Candida in its harmless form is present in small numbers in the normal gut. But it always has the potential to become pathogenic - that is, become capable of causing disease. Within the intestine it's controlled by a healthy environment. If the balance in favour of the friendly organisms is lost - which happens in a variety of ways that we'll go into in the chapter 'From Genes to Jeans' - candida can increase alarmingly, either causing the mast cells to degranulate or by developing long root-like structures that penetrate the gut wall. Either way, candida can circulate to any part of the body and manifests itself as a fungus, thrush being, perhaps, the best-known of its unsavoury forms. Once converted into its pathogenic form, candida can go wild, multiplying at a phenomenal rate, burrowing into tissues and joints - and, in the process, making the sufferer feel sick all over. Given the perfect environment candida organisms multiply so fast they could in theory cover the world; however, as a new colony develops on top of an old one, the latter dies from lack of food.

In common with most yeasts, candida feeds on sugar - and human beings run on glucose as surely as cars run on petrol. Someone with candida in their bloodstream is essentially eating for it as well as for themselves. Candida loves sugar and when it wants more it forces your blood-sugar levels down alarmingly, making you crave carbohydrate.

Once that wouldn't have had any particular repercussion: in a "pre-processed" world the only carbohydrates available were grains and natural fruits, which delivered their sugar in a very slow and gentle way. Today, modern methods of food manufacture provide a mass of refined carbohydrates - chocolate bars, biscuits, doughnuts, white bread - which the body absorbs too easily and which rapidly raise the blood sugar - thereby providing candida with a plentiful supply of what it desires.

If the candida eats the sugar, why should you put on weight? The answer is, in responding to the craving that the candida has induced, you don't just eat enough to make you feel satisfied, you tend to overdo it, so raising your blood sugar far more than you need - and far more than the candida needs. That makes your body fire off insulin to bring down your blood sugar into the normal range, which it does by pushing the sugar out of the bloodstream and depositing it as fat in the tissues. The more the insulin mechanism is called into play, the more sugar is deposited as fat. Because of their eating habits, many people swing from a high blood sugar to a low many times a day. In some, this finally exhausts the insulin-making mechanism - leading to adult onset diabetes. Diabetics produce too little insulin and have to inject it, as well as avoiding foods that release a lot of glucose at once - sugar and other sweet foods. Adult onset diabetes is on the increase in this country.

How widespread is candida? In 'The Yeast Syndrome' Doctor John Trowbridge surmised that it affects one-third of the total populations of Western industrialised countries - a view supported by many researchers. Candidiasis, however, is rarely diagnosed - the symptoms of candidiasis appear as separate illnesses and are "treated" with palliatives, to the detriment of sufferers' health.

Hypoglycaemia - low blood sugar - is, more often than not, candida's partner in crime (it's possible to have low blood sugar without having candida). It occurs when the body, faced with an onslaught of high-glucose foods, produces a large amount of insulin to drive down the blood sugar. Because the Western world is addicted to sugar and refined carbohydrate, "normal" blood-sugar levels are higher than they should be. In general terms few symptoms result from moderately raised blood sugar - although excessive levels make a person thirsty and can do a lot of damage to blood vessels in the long run - whereas many symptoms occur when blood sugar levels fall too low - sweating, palpitations, even loss of consciousness. Hyperactive children are often victims of hypoglycaemia. And, again, the cause of the low blood sugar that brings on their symptoms - their inability to keep still, concentrate or finish anything they start, their tendency to talk too fast, their tantrums - is food intolerance.

Talking about "low" blood sugar is misleading. What counts is the severity of the drop. The effect on your body of whizzing from medium to low is precisely the same as from high to medium and your body reacts in precisely the same way - it craves something sweet. When it does and you feed it, the scenario we've described under candida unreels.

Do you feel irritated if you're late for a meal? Are you sometimes going happily about your business - doing the shopping, picking up the kids from school, cleaning the car - when suddenly you feel light-headed or weak or anxious and your heart is thumping? Does your concentration suddenly go in the middle of something important? And do the symptoms disappear when you eat - preferably something sugary - but return after an hour or so?

You are undoubtedly hypoglycaemic - exactly the kind of person who gets nowhere with calorie counting because, however faithfully you stay under your calorie ceiling, you include foods that create the hypoglycaemic situation. People with severe hypoglycaemic conditions even have to take food to bed with them and seem to spend their life within chewing distance of the fridge.

It's most unlikely that anyone with a weight problem is not a victim of at least one of the three conditions we've described. And, as we'll continue to repeat, they all stem from food intolerance.

* * *

Why food intolerance occurs is not yet understood, or why different foods go "rogue" in different people. Its existence began to be known at the end of the last century. There is a highly respected corpus of work on the subject, even in books popular enough to be found on public library shelves. But because the only way of testing people has been case by case, by the slow, laborious and inconsistent method of trial and error - and because work in this field has largely been carried out by scientists outside the medical mainstream and has been used by doctors and nutritionists who've tended not to conform to medical orthodoxy - the subject has not aroused the commercial interest which developments in any sphere require to get them off the ground. While the public has gradually become aware of food intolerance, notably in relation to long-term illness, the subject has stayed on the fringes of medicine.

Much of the information we've given you about food intolerance is openly available, if not as widely as it might be. The reasons for that are understandable: while the public at large has always been eager (even gullibly eager) to try other methods of weight loss which books and magazines bring to their attention, the "orthodox" view of the importance of calories has remained entrenched. And, it's fair to say, having failed to understand that, in practical terms, reducing calorie intake below the energy requirement is unsustainable for any reasonable period without ill-health, the public has been unwilling to listen to the lone voices which from time to time have said anything to the contrary.

Yet one study has shown that, on very low-calorie diets - on which people certainly can lose weight - the drop-out rate is 93%. We might add that it hasn't been in the interests of either the manufacturers of "healthy" low-calorie foods and drinks or the multi-million-pound dieting industry to change the public's perception.

For years, some informed medical practitioners have treated the overweight, as well as those suffering from chronic conditions, by removing their food intolerances, usually by employing some form of elimination diet. This takes a patient off everything but water for a number of days to clear the system, though sometimes a handful of what are hoped to be "safe" foods are allowed during this period. Foods are then re-introduced to the diet singly and indications of an adverse reaction to each one looked for - a slow, inaccurate and painfully uncomfortable method. What was needed to drag food intolerance, the villain of overweight, into the centre of the stage - and kick the hero-impostor, the theory of calorie counting, into the wings - was a test procedure that was quick, accurate and capable of dealing with large numbers of people.

We have developed such a procedure. It has taken us two years. It achieves the kind of weight loss which until now you could only have dreamed of. And we have proved it works using a benchmark test accepted by the medical profession.

WE HAVE CALLED THE PROCEDURE THE NUTRON DIET. IN THE SENSE THAT PEOPLE UNDERSTAND DIETING, NO DIET IS INVOLVED. AND THE NUTRON DIET MAKES EVERY OTHER WEIGHT-LOSS DIET OBSOLETE.

DISCOVERING HOW TO DO IT
part one

Patrick Kingsley's philosophy of medicine is that illness is a symptom not a cause and that doctors who treat symptoms are not treating patients. Anyone used to seeing their GP on the in-out conveyor belt of a general practice would be staggered to be seen by Doctor Kingsley for the first time. New patients spend seventy-five minutes with him; other consultations are an hour. He wants to know everything about a patient. Not just their medical details. Everything. "Without knowing someone's personal history, treatment is guesswork," he says.

For over two decades he's believed that food intolerance is the cause of being overweight.

A neat, slim man of fifty-five who rides, plays tennis and is a Midlands regional hockey umpire, Patrick Kingsley is a familiar figure on his daily run around the Leicestershire village where he lives. While a student in London during the 1960s, he earned money to help keep himself by appearing as an extra in innumerable British films including 'A Tale of Two Cities', 'Dunkirk', 'The Captain's Table', 'The Yellow Rolls-Royce', and half-a-dozen James Bond movies. Usually he was just one of the crowd, but if someone was needed to drive a roadster or ride a horse he often got the part. Occasionally he even had a few lines. He also did some modelling and appeared in over two hundred television commercials. Most medical students are hard up;

he drove a twin-cam MGA.

Patrick Kingsley's professional career became at least as distinguished as his looks. He set up the clinical pharmacology department of the international chemical giant Fisons, dealing with a range of world-wide research projects. With three other doctors he founded the British Society for Nutritional Medicine, later merged with the British Society for Allergy and Environmental Medicine. He is Chief Medical Officer of Foresight (The Association for Promotion of Preconceptual Care), a Fellow of the American Academy of Environmental Medicine, a published author, lecturer and broadcaster.

During the eight years he was at Fisons, Patrick Kingsley took up a post as Honorary Clinical Assistant in the Department of Allergy at Nottingham City Hospital. One day he came to treat a woman who developed an urticarial rash (hives) whenever she ate citrus fruit of any kind; even a small amount of lemon juice as seasoning affected her. If she ate fish she was vomiting for the next twenty-four hours.

At the time, Patrick Kingsley was involved at Fisons with a new drug called Intal, which prevented asthmatic attacks when taken by inhalation. It occurred to him that if Intal could prevent an asthmatic attack, it might also prevent his patient's symptoms if she took the drug by mouth before eating the foods that made her ill. He tried it and it worked*

---

* Kingsley. P.J., 'Sodium Cromoglycate in Gastro-intestinal Allergy.' The Lancet, 2: 1011, 1974.

But why? He traced the chemical pathway to a conclusion. In asthmatics, the drug desensitised the mast cells in the lungs, preventing them from releasing the harmful chemicals that cause the symptoms; in his patient, it had acted in a similar way on the intestinal mast cells, effectively stopping her reacting to her intolerant foods.

In the early 1970s, hardly anyone in this country knew anything about how people react against food, with the notable exception of Dr Richard Mackarness, a psychiatrist at Basingstoke District Hospital who'd opened the first clinical ecology unit in Britain, where he'd introduced the use of an elimination diet he'd learnt in America. Patrick Kingsley went to see him and concluded that clinical ecology - which is the study of man's reaction to everything in his environment - had much to teach orthodox medicine.

The orthodox approach to all disease is that the organ that's showing symptoms is where the problem lies. The approach of clinical ecology is that something in the organ's environment has caused it to react; removing the cause - which is often a reaction against food - makes the symptoms disappear.

Patrick Kingsley later spent time training in clinical ecology in Canada. Then, first in general and then private practice, he continued to treat as many patients as possible using an holistic approach, frequently employing the eradication of food intolerances. Right from the beginning he was aware that clinical success in many disorders was often accompanied by significant weight loss.

Although he used several methods throughout the 1980s, Patrick Kingsley favoured the five-day fast to identify food intolerance. As the name implies, anyone undergoing this treatment could eat nothing during it, living on spring or bottled water. After five days, foods were re-introduced one by one, with the patient having to record their weight several times a day, keep notes on their consumption and write down their observations of their reactions.

The method worked, perhaps most dramatically with two women whom he happened, coincidentally, to treat about the same time. Both were middle-aged and unknown to each other. Mrs P weighed nineteen-and-a-half stone, Miss T eighteen-and-a-half stone. Both had been to various slimming clubs in the area, both were now on a 500-calorie diet and both, to their horror, had actually gained weight while adhering to it.

In five days' fasting, Mrs P lost twenty-one pounds, Miss T eighteen pounds. On the second stage of the treatment, when the orderly re-introduction of foods began, both put on nearly three-quarters of a stone in twenty-four hours - at which point Doctor Kingsley found out they were intolerant to carrots, with Mrs P additionally intolerant to cabbage and Miss T to cauliflower - three items not surprisingly recommended in their low-calorie diet. Once these foods (and certain others that produced less dramatic effects) were removed from their menu, both women steadily lost stones in weight, which did not return. And the symptoms both suffered, including apathy, headaches and fatigue, left them.

The massive weight loss which Mrs P and Miss T experienced merely underlined Patrick Kingsley's conviction that accumulated fluid was masquerading as fat. Fluid, caused by food intolerance, was responsible for a significant amount of overweight conditions. But, as he knew only too well, this flew in the face of accepted medical belief and the conventional wisdom of the dieting business which said - and continues to say - that only a small percentage of overweight is due to fluid retention.

For there to be any chance of changing that thinking, an automated test that could incontrovertibly demonstrate otherwise had to be found. The story went on hold until 1991.

* * *

Ian Stoakes first met Patrick Kingsley in 1985, when at the age of thirty-one he became fund-raiser for the British Society for Nutritional Medicine and immediately found himself fascinated by the older man's work. Despite his mainstream credentials - Bart's, the Royal College of Surgeons, the Royal College of Obstetricians and Gynaecologists - Patrick Kingsley was someone, Ian Stoakes felt, who looked beyond the narrow confines of orthodoxy. By now, Doctor Kingsley was treating multiple sclerosis sufferers on the basis of food intolerance, but he was also prepared to experiment with the removal of amalgam teeth fillings which lodges mercury poisoning in the spinal fluid of MS sufferers. Many of his patients were coming to him in advanced stages of their condition, confined to wheelchairs, but he was achieving a significant level of success in making them well. "When I saw what he was doing," Ian Stoakes says simply, "I was dedicated to him for life."

Why Patrick Kingsley took to the fast-talking younger man was because he got things done, never stopped asking questions, and always had an alternative point of view - and he had already amassed a considerable knowledge about nutrition. "Ian has the most remarkably inquiring mind and he can explain science in the exciting way scientists can't," he observes. "He can make associations that don't occur to other people. And he can clarify a complex topic, not only for ordinary people but for scientists of different disciplines who have no idea how to talk to each other."

* * *

There was nothing orthodox about Ian Stoakes' career. After leaving Christ Church College, he'd become the deputy principal of a training unit for mentally handicapped adolescents in Kent, where he'd tried to introduce the idea that it was possible to alter behaviour through diet. Because the cook refused to prepare individual meals, he resigned, moving to Slough as the youngest principal of a Home Office secure unit, which housed adolescents convicted of violent crime. Here he extended the ways of investigating and changing behaviour patterns, retaining his interest in the part played by diet.

In the two years that he then worked for the British Society for Nutritional Medicine, Ian Stoakes came to believe that what Patrick Kingsley and others working in the nutritional field were doing was right. Many conversations between the two men circled the same subject. That what food intolerance cried out for was a credible test: one which was quick, accurate, free of operator involvement, and was at least relatively cheap.

In 1989, Ian Stoakes became chief executive of the Dietary Research Foundation, running a multi-national two-year study, conducted on both sides of the Atlantic, which in various ways involved double Nobel Laureate Linus Pauling and Professors John Yudkin and Hans Eysenck. One part of the study was directed towards changing the behaviour of juvenile delinquents by reducing their intake of empty calories; the other measured the effects on children's intellectual development by adding nutrients to their diet.

As the study was winding down, two things happened which helped make the breakthrough that food intolerance needed: Ian Stoakes was asked to help promote a Yorkshire clinic that was treating disease by testing for food intolerance - and he got an agonising pain in his back.

The clinic was using the cytotoxic (it means cell poison) test, which mixed a blood sample with food extracts that were viewed on slides through a microscope. Published studies have shown the test to be 70-90% reliable when carried out under strict conditions but, while a major advance on the five-day fast, it depended on the expertise of an operator who was checking some seventy slides - a procedure that slowed as the laboratory technician tired. The clinic could deal with only twenty cases a day.

What caught Ian Stoakes' eye was that many of the clinic's patients, while reporting huge improvement in their well-being, were also reporting considerable weight loss. It seemed obvious to him that the clinic should promote itself as providing a radical way of slimming and he put out a press release. The result was a double-page spread in the 'Daily Express', seven thousand inquiries in five weeks and bookings that stretched from summer to Christmas. Blood samples were flown in from the Arab Emirates on private jets, they came from France, one sample arrived at the door in a Rolls-Royce.

The clinic could not cope with the demand: some means of automation had to be found. At first Ian Stoakes thought it might be possible to set up a system whereby a TV camera the size of a pencil could be attached to the microscope and linked to a computer to analyse the results instead of an operator. Then - out of the blue - he thought: why not use a haematology analyser - the kind of machine used in hospital pathology departments up and down the land? If an analyser could process blood, why not blood and food extract? He got on to an American manufacturer and persuaded them to give him the use of a machine.

The outcome wasn't encouraging. While the machine was capable of analysing a blood and food mix, it clogged rapidly and repeatedly, necessitating hours of stripping down and cleaning. The problem seemed insoluble.

At this point, in one of those ironies of fate, Ian Stoakes was laid low with a back pain so acute he could only stand by bracing himself up his bedroom wall. For two weeks he lived with the possibility that he had renal failure. Then a cytotoxic test showed he was intolerant to milk, he stopped taking it - and the pain went away. And he went back to trying to solve the problem of the haematology analyser. For a time he toyed with the possibility of a purpose-built machine, but that would have needed considerable capital outlay (an off-the-shelf machine costs in the region of £100,000). The clinic was unwilling to contemplate that kind of investment. It and Ian Stoakes parted company.

Did all analysers behave in the same way or was it possible that a differently made machine might not clog? In his ebullient fashion, Ian Stoakes believes that the answer to any problem can't be more than three phone-calls away. Quickly he found that Toa, a Japanese manufacturer, had just opened an office in Britain, at Milton Keynes. He called them. "How many machines do you sell in Britain a year?" he asked. Thirty, he was told. "How would you like to sell hundreds?" he asked.

Toa sent a delegation to see him the next day. After some encouraging negotiations it was agreed that he would go to Milton Keynes to run the test. It was his own blood mixed with milk extract that went through the haematology analyser a short time later. The Japanese were polite, helpful - and sceptical. But, even if Ian Stoakes' heart was in his mouth, he felt sure the experiment would work; the very fact that his food intolerance had surfaced when it had was surely a sign. He watched the screen. The American machine had worked on a different display principle which was nothing like the big, bright computer graphics that were now in front of him, showing in a three-dimensional scattergram what the machine was doing. Suddenly some of the white dots that represented the white cells in the sample appeared to undergo a disturbance. "The machine's malfunctioned," someone said.

Had it? A member of Toa's staff volunteered to give a blood sample, this was mixed with milk and went through the machine. Now there was no disturbance - clearly something different had happened when Ian Stoakes' intolerance was present. What? For the moment that didn't matter. "It was," he says, "a true eureka moment."

It didn't, in fact, take long to find out what had happened. The neutrophils in Ian Stoakes' blood sample, degranulated by his known milk intolerance, had appeared to the haematology analyser to have taken on the characteristics of monocytes, another of the while cell group. The machine had duly counted them as such - with the scattergram visually recording this as if the damaged neutrophils had physically moved from one cluster to another. It was as simple as that.

Just as importantly - the Toa machine didn't clog, however

30

many tests were run through it.

Ian Stoakes went to see a senior professor at a London teaching hospital to find out if there was any test against which the breakthrough could be measured. No, there was nothing. But the advice couldn't have been plainer: "If what you're doing works on people it's a good procedure. If it doesn't, it's back to the drawing-board."

* * *

part two

We began to use the test on patients at the practice. For reasons we've explained, the test was just as significant in the treatment of many illnesses as well as in controlling weight. By working with people who were fairly ill, and with others who were fairly ill and overweight, we were able to monitor the effects on both illness and weight loss. Many of the results of the treatment of a number of medical conditions were staggering. *But the weight loss many people experienced was no less staggering, with some casting off stones.*

Patients taking part in the experiment had only to give a blood sample - which many, sadly, were only too familiar with doing - and then change their diet in the ways that we asked them. In all instances it involved excluding certain foods and in keeping to certain others. In some cases we substituted foods for those to which different patients showed an intolerance. Many actually enjoyed this aspect - as one said, eating different foods was what she only got to do on holiday!

Initially, we ran the test in a limited way, using thirty staple items. It was during this period that we approached a women's slimming club and asked if the members could take part in a controlled experiment. The owner agreed, the members gave their blood samples, received their diets, eliminated the foods to which their bodies reacted and shed pounds in sensational fashion. Everyone was delighted - until the owner realised something which, in all honesty, we hadn't thought through. We were likely to put her out of business. She called the experiment to a halt, denying that it had worked or that her members had lost weight - although angry women were ringing us up telling us this wasn't true. Among them was one very overweight woman who had not only dropped several stones but who'd begun to find that the arthritis from which she'd suffered for twenty years - so badly that she couldn't lift her leg sufficiently to step up and down from the pavement - had begun to vanish. (We've kept in touch with her and nearly two years later her arthritis has virtually gone.)

The episode, we're sorry to say, ended in shambles. But for us it had been the first major demonstration of what the test and diet could do for a group of ordinary women who wanted to be slimmer - and it had brought home to us something we've already told you: *that what we were doing made every other way of slimming redundant.*

What we now had to decide was how many foods it was practicable to test.

Food extracts began to be manufactured for skin-prick allergy testing - a field closely related to food intolerance. More than three hundred foods are available in extract form - pulverised, freeze-dried, added to distilled water and filtered, a process which is conducted in "polished air" conditions of hygiene. But the more of them we included, the more expensive the test would become - and it was important that The NuTron Diet was affordable. In the end we settled on about a third of the available number, which included all the items anyone is likely to eat and which also made commercial sense.

THE NUTRON DIET

* * *

The medical profession at large is understandably sceptical of any cure or treatment that has not been exposed to the benchmark test which is called the double-blind placebo controlled trial. That is a terrible mouthful, but the basis of it is simple. A placebo is a dummy, a harmless substitute for the cure or treatment that's actually under scrutiny but which is indistinguishable from it. A placebo test usually involves two groups of people, one of which gets the dummy while the other gets the real thing. After an agreed period comes the cross-over - the groups are swapped round for a similar period, not knowing whether they're moving from the placebo to the treatment, or vice-versa.

By July 1993, some four hundred people had been through our procedure and we'd perfected it to the point where we could have put it before the public. We chose not to do that - because we wanted to expose our beliefs to an independent placebo test. There was a risk involved in this decision. We were confident that The NuTron Diet did everything we said it did. If, however, it failed the placebo test, ethically and morally we would have come to the end of the road.

A five-doctor group practice in the Home Counties, where one of the partners had an interest in food intolerance, agreed to conduct the trial, using twenty volunteers from its patient list, all of them excessively overweight. The protocol was approved by the Ethics Committee of the local Health Authority. If twenty sounds an insignificant number of people to use in such a critically important study, that isn't so. As one of Britain's leading epidemiologists has said, a large number of "guinea-pigs" is only necessary in a trial that's attempting to determine a small shift of some sort; where a massive swing is being looked for, only a small number is required - and we were looking for big weight losses...

Having taken the volunteers' blood samples and recorded their food intolerances, the practice took over. The fate of The NuTron Diet had now moved beyond our control.

The manner in which the study was carried out, as we'd agreed it with the practice, was standard. Half the volunteers were put on The NuTron Diet, with all the foods to which each was intolerant removed. The other half were given the placebo diet, with an equivalent number of foods taken out but with the "intolerant" foods left in. After ten days, the groups changed diets for another period of ten days. There were no restrictions on either menu - the participants were encouraged to eat what they liked and as much as they liked to the limit of their appetite.

Confidence is one thing, waiting another - and three weeks is a long time to wait. But then we were given the results. In the ten days each group had been on The NuTron Diet, the average weight loss had been half a stone - with one participant losing over a stone. Significantly, the group which had been on The NuTron Diet first, had begun to put weight back on once they'd gone over to the placebo diet which contained the foods to which they were intolerant. Just as significantly, the placebo group had not experienced any weight loss until they transferred to The NuTron Diet.

For the first time in history, as far as we know, a diet for the public at large had been subjected to a double-blind placebo cross-over. And it had come through with flying colours.

* * *

If you want to put yourself on The NuTron Diet, how do you go about it?

The first thing is to have a sample of your blood taken. It doesn't matter where you live: the sample can be drawn locally and sent to the laboratory for analysis; but it's important that it's drawn by someone who is suitably experienced, which in most cases will be your GP, or practice nurse. In view of the part which The NuTron Diet can play in the treatment of many illnesses, it may well be of value to the doctor to know anyway - he or she can keep an eye on any medical condition a dieter may have, with a view to altering treatment.

Clients must use the special Vacutainer pack that is provided, which includes two 10ml vials containing the anti-coagulant, sodium citrate.

Once, having a blood sample taken was a disagreeable business - needles used time and again were frequently blunt, there was the unpleasant sensation of the manual piston of the syringe drawing the blood, as often as not accompanied by an equally unpleasant noise, and often an ugly raised lump was left behind, surrounded by bruising. Sometimes patients became so distressed they suffered collapsed veins, which made drawing a sample impossible.

The Vacutainer system has changed all that. No syringe is involved, merely an adapter, about the diameter of a biro refill and half its length. This is used only once and its needle is so fine and so sharp that it slips into the vein rather than puncturing it. Only when the cap of one of the vials is pierced by the end opposite to the needle is the vacuum which draws the blood engaged. The second vial is filled in the same way, without the needle having to be withdrawn and reinserted. The entire procedure takes painless seconds.

A sample must be drawn on the day preceding the test. Blood taken from the body is "alive" for only twenty-four hours, but the forward-booking system that's been put in place, and an arrangement with a nation-wide carrier for collection and overnight delivery, ensure that a sample is received in less than that time.

Once the 20ml sample arrives at the laboratory, it's divided into ninety-six sub-samples. Four are mixed with a diluent (a simple saline solution), ninety-one with food extracts - and one with a candida extract. All ninety-six are then placed in the tiny wells of a tray measuring twelve wells across by eight down - each about a third of the size of a thimble. It's important that every blood sample and every blood-and-extract mixture goes into a specific well - the haematology analyser's computer matches the analysis of each well to its numbered position for read-out.

A tray of blood and food extracts is ready for analysis after a carefully controlled incubation period.

Three of the five groups of white blood cells - the eosinophils, the basophils and the neutrophils - are, as we've told you, granulocytes: that is, they have in their make-up the toxic "marbles" we've talked about. As the eosinophils and basophils constitute less than five percent of the granulocytes, they are ignored for the purposes of testing.

First, the haematology analyser "reads" the four sub-samples of blood and diluant, establishing both the state of the neutrophils and their number. These readings are averaged to give the base-line against which the readings from the other sub-samples will be measured.

The analyser takes thirty seconds to test each sample. What it's looking to see is whether during incubation any extract - and, in one case, the candida organism - has attacked the neutrophils. It does this by interrogating each neutrophil cell by passing radio frequency pulses through it and direct current pulses around it. If the cells are undamaged, the number of neutrophils in the sample equals the number established as the base-line - there is no intolerance. If, however, there is damage, the machine measures this both in absolute numbers and as a percentage and records the proportion of damaged neutrophils as monocytes - one of the two groups of white blood cells which don't contain toxic "marbles".

A print-out of every NuTron Test involves complex data and is scrutinised by a nurse-practitioner to ensure nutritional adequacy. Only when he or she is satisfied that the readings are accurate will they be passed so that another linked computer can generate a client's individual diet. If something suspicious *were* revealed by a print-out, which could happen if, for instance, a blood sample reached the laboratory later than twenty-four hours after being drawn and the cells had begun to die, we would abort the test and ask for another sample. That would be rare - but it's important that you know we've built in such a safeguard.

From first to last NuTron analysis takes an hour. *It is probably the single most important hour of any dieter's life* - because the individual diet that results from it holds the key to their body's future.

Is it possible that you won't lose weight by following The NuTron Diet? Of course it is. Your body is a complicated piece of machinery and you may have other problems which prevent weight loss; or you may not give enough attention to what we're saying about what you should and shouldn't eat. One client who was intolerant to wheat failed to lose even a few pounds and told us indignantly that he'd observed his diet religiously - except, we discovered, that he snacked repeatedly on Penguin bars without considering what their biscuit base was made of.

Unquestionably the vast majority of people who've followed The NuTron Diet have regarded it an unqualified success. Not only have they lost weight - spectacularly in cases of severe overweight - but they've done it while leading their normal lives. Most have also found their general well-being and zest for living increase.

The NuTron Diet isn't too simple to be true - it is simply true. And unlike any popular diet, it's preventative as well as curative.

All it takes to be slim is adherence to two rules: avoid the foods to which you are intolerant; eat from the foods to which you know you're not intolerant. AND WITHIN THAT FRAMEWORK YOU CAN EAT TO YOUR APPETITE, FORGET THE CALORIE COUNTER AND THE BATHROOM SCALES AND REACH FOR THE TRACKSUIT OR THE LEOTARD ONLY IN PURSUIT OF GREATER FITNESS AND PLEASURE.

THERE IS LIFE AFTER TESTING

On average, people taking The NuTron Test are intolerant to between ten and fifteen foods. Clare Hickman found she reacted to twenty-five. "When I got my results, I knew the foods I'd have to avoid would be in red and the foods that were safe for me would be in green," she says. "As I drew the sheet from the envelope, the red list went on and on. I didn't even look at the green. I just thought: 'I might as well die, there isn't anything I can eat.'"

Clare is thirty-two, a mother of four, and she wants to lose twelve pounds. At five feet seven she's nine stone eleven and doesn't look overweight because she's small framed, but she's aware of the excess on her stomach and hips. What galls her is that, with one son who's hyperactive, a baby who won't sleep, and a husband who often works nights, she doesn't even get time to eat regularly.

When she married she was just over eight stone, but she's had increasing trouble getting her weight down after the birth of each of her children and it's a constant battle to keep it where it is. She's a former medical secretary with some knowledge of nutrition and she's been on a number of diets without lasting success. And, even though she thinks there's something in the claims of The NuTron Diet, she's still just a bit cynical.

Clare took her test at around midday on Wednesday. It was now 8am Friday and she stood disconsolately looking into the fridge, crossing off in her mind the things she could no longer have. "Then I spotted the sliced ham - that wasn't on my banned list. So I nibbled a slice and tried to console myself."

Over three thousand people have been through The NuTron Test and only two or three have had no reaction against any of the list of ninety-two foods. Many have reacted to only one or two foods, but we've had clients intolerant to over fifty. Clare's twenty-six was higher than average but by no means abnormal and we're telling you her story for a number of reasons: because she's too forthright to be anything but honest; because she's the average dieter - most women who are not excessively overweight still want to lose between half a stone and a stone; and because it's easier to show how the principles of The NuTron Diet work when they're applied to one individual.

These are the foods to which Clare tested intolerantly, in *descending* order of reaction:

Baker's yeast
Malt
Brewer's yeast
Chilli pepper
Coffee
Milk whey
Mushroom
Coconut
Cheese
Black pepper
Gluten
Spinach
Egg white
Curry powder
Tomato

Tannin (includes
 tea,
red wine,
 plum,
raisin,
currant)
Radish

Candida reaction
(therefore avoid chocolate,
melon*, sugar cane, sugar
beet)
* Melon is to be avoided because,
unlike other fruits, it moulds
from the inside - and candida is
itself a mould

41

THE NUTRON DIET

But this is the *other* list which Clare received, from which she could make her meals:

Meats
Beef
Chicken
Lamb
Pork
Rabbit
Turkey

Fish
Cod
Crab
Haddock
Halibut
Herring
Mackerel
Salmon
Shrimp
Sole
Trout
Tuna

Dairy
Egg yolk

Vegetables
Aubergine
Baked Bean
Broccoli
Brussels sprout
Cabbage
Carrot
Cauliflower
Courgette
Garlic
Lentil
Parsnip
Pea
Potato
Runner bean
Soya bean
Turnip

Salads
Beetroot
Celery
Cucumber
Bell pepper
Lettuce
Onion

Misc
White pepper
Salt

Fruit
Apple
Banana
Grape white
Grapefruit
Lemon
Mango
Orange
Olive
Peach
Pear
Pineapple
Raspberry
Rhubarb
Strawberry

Grains
Barley
Corn*
Oats
Rice

Nuts
Almond
Brazil
Peanut
Sesame seed*
Sunflower seed*
Walnut

* Including oils

Once over her initial disbelief, Clare began to realise this second list was pretty comprehensive - and that a couple of items on her banned list, namely spinach and radish, were things she didn't even like or eat. Reducing the number mentally made her feel better. "But I was still thinking about all the things I couldn't eat and couldn't drink," she says. "Then I suddenly cheered up for the silly reason that it occurred to me I hadn't tested intolerant to apples. I live on apples. If they'd been on the banned side with everything else, I really think I might have given up before I started. But they weren't and I felt that was a lucky sign."

Sitting at her dining-room table that Friday morning, she set her own small test by which she would judge the success of The NuTron Diet. She hadn't been able to take off her wedding ring since her first pregnancy in 1985, eight years previously, when her fingers had fattened around the knuckles. If she could do that, she thought, then she'd admit the diet had worked...

* * *

Why does anyone suffer from food intolerance?

We know that a diet stuffed full of sugar and refined carbohydrate is a principle cause of overweight. But does it cause food intolerance? For the time being no-one knows and we can only speculate; as we can about the stress of modern life as a cause; or the chemicals and pollutants we can't avoid taking into our bodies just by living in the world as it is today - and for which our physiology, when it was developing two million years ago, was never designed. And what about the part played by genetics? Possibly people's genetic code stores a pre-disposition to intolerance - as we've emphasised, everybody is an individual: even identical twins have tested intolerant to different foods.

But in the final analysis, the causes don't matter. Food intolerance exists. It is a regular phenomenon. And if you are overweight, it's quite likely due to food intolerance.

In a vague way, people have been aware of food intolerance for a very long time - as allergies. In fact, there are important differences between intolerances and allergies though many doctors seemingly are unaware of them.

An allergy is an over-reaction of the body's defence mechanism caused by a substance with which the sufferer doesn't normally come into contact, or eat. To challenge this substance (called an antigen), the body creates immunoglobulins (Ig), one type of which, the IgE, is of especial importance. The classic allergic reaction is near-immediate and easy to recognise - an asthma attack while visiting someone who has a cat; the outbreak of a rash after eating strawberries. Some allergies - notably an allergy to peanuts - can kill. *Food intolerances, on the other hand, don't involve IgE - and most intolerant reactions develop slowly and stealthily, tending to involve common foods that are eaten frequently.*

None of this is important to you other than in setting the record straight. You'll have heard of people being allergic to certain foods when what was meant was that they were food intolerant. And you'll have heard of people having such an "allergy" to something as broad-based as "dairy produce". This, as The NuTron Test demonstrates, is a blanket judgement - food intolerances are usually very much more specific. Clare, for instance, tested intolerantly to the whey in milk - but not to the lactose; and to egg white - but not egg yolk. In other words, The NuTron Test won't decimate your diet - just pluck out the problems.

44

Taking the test is the first step towards identifying those problems. Clare was now taking the second step - coming to terms with her individual NuTron Diet.

Her initial reaction on reading her banned list had been panic. Almost all our clients tell us the same thing - and that the panic is accompanied by a feeling of disbelief. But at least Clare could keep her favourite apples; the majority of clients find their favourite food is on their intolerant list. Having said that, a lot of people who are addicted to chocolate and expect to find they're intolerant to it, test negatively - *but lose their addiction when they come off the foods to which they're actually intolerant.*

The reason, as we told you in Chapter One, is simple: once the body gets back into balance it's no longer looking for that quick carbohydrate fix.

And Clare had begun to think positively - which is our first message in making The NuTron Diet work. Things could be worse. Imagine what it was like, before The NuTron Diet became possible, submitting yourself to an elimination diet - which was the only semi-reliable way of establishing what your intolerances were. Starvation, or near-starvation, for days. Then the single re-introduction of foods into your diet until you noted an adverse reaction - which prompted the removal of the offending item from your intake. And so on, until the next adverse reaction. What an unpleasant, not to say inaccurate, way of finding out, over what could be months, what The NuTron Test can tell you effortlessly, accurately and immediately!

Our second message, to reiterate something we told you in the previous chapter: the diet isn't really about what you *can't* eat, it's about what you *can* - without setting off the cycle of intolerance that leads to weight gain. Don't worry about the things that have to come off your menu. Concentrate on the eighty or so foods that The NuTron Diet indicates ARE SAFE FOR YOU.

Our third message is given with a bit of a smile flickering around our lips: don't "dare" one of your food intolerances to do its worst.

Actually, we know it's almost not worth giving you this advice. Once The NuTron Diet begins to work you'll start to think that your weight loss can't *really* be because you've given up something like coffee or cheese. And you'll take a cup or two, or a slice or two - defiantly. And you'll get the mother of all headaches and put back possibly half a stone overnight. And, too late, you'll remember that we told you so...

* * *

Clare has written down what she's been used to eating.

Pizza, chilli con carne, curry, garlic bread, cheese pie, biscuits and cheese (cheddar, brie, cottage), a bowl of milk and cereal at night. And endless sandwiches instead of proper meals, as well as the usual cake and sweet biscuit nibbles. All have brought her intolerances into play, as has the percolated coffee and cream that she drinks constantly, the hot chocolate, the hot yeast extract, the "nightcap" drinks, the lager, the red wine.

Because of her intolerance to gluten and baker's yeast, Clare can't have bread or pastry in any form, but even if she hadn't tested positively to these we'd have advised her to avoid them anyway, because of her candida reaction. As we've indicated, the body treats refined carbohydrates as if they were sugar and anyone showing a candida reaction should avoid sugar of every kind, as well as foods and drinks which involve yeasts in the manufacturing process and foods of the mould type such as mushrooms and cheese. As it happens, because of the particular spread of Clare's intolerances, all these things are already on her banned list. By removing them from her diet, the candida within her intestines will be starved.

Clare's been paying more attention to her green list, which gives her the all-clear for all the meats, all the fish and all the fruits (with the exception of melon because of her candida reaction). Gluten has knocked out barley, oats, rye and wheat, but she's still left with corn and rice.

"I now don't feel restricted by my diet, I realise the number of meals I can prepare from the safe list is very wide," she says. "But I also realise I'm going to have to get the children used to some different things, too. Like most mothers I tend to eat whatever the children are eating and I don't want to put temptation in my way."

She's come back from Tesco's with three boxes of rice cakes to substitute for her morning toast, soya milk, and a lot of fresh fish which she hadn't been in the habit of buying. She'd thought fish was expensive and is surprised it's less so than she expected: whole boned kipper for 44p, whole mackerel for 99p, smoked cod at £1.60 a pound. She's also brought back a carton of sugar-free, caffeine-free Coke.

As someone who tends to take a hot drink rather than eat, Clare says that at first she was more concerned about what the diet was going to do to her liquid rather than her solid intake - it seemed to leave her nothing at all. She feels a bit foolish about that now - she has the Coke, she can choose from any of the fruit concentrates which she can also have hot/diluted, and she's taken to hot water with a squeeze of lemon. And she isn't intolerant to white wine - though, as yeast goes into its production, she intends to avoid it for the first month, because of her candida reaction.

Two days into her diet, she rings her parents to say

that the baby has slept through the night for the first time in his six-and-a-half month life; usually Dominic has her up every two hours. On the following day he sleeps for three-and-a-half hours during the day, never before having gone as long as an hour.

As we said earlier, Clare is cynical about diets and can't - yet - say she's completely confident that The NuTron Diet works. But would she agree that, as she's still breast feeding, it's at least possible Dominic is now sleeping better because she's no longer passing her food intolerances on?

"I'm aware that pregnant women who smoke can pass on their addiction to babies in the womb. So perhaps my percolated coffee had been keeping Dominic awake. But it's just as possible that at this age he might have started sleeping through, anyway. It could be coincidence."

In the two days Clare loses four pounds.

On the third day, she awakes to another two pound loss but with what feels like flu: a dull headache, aching joints, a blocked nose. But the notes she was sent with her NuTron Test results have told her this is usual - she's got withdrawal symptoms. Dominic has again slept through the night and again for over three hours in the afternoon. Clare should be pleased but she's grumpy: and gets grumpier later in the morning when she's vacuuming. Pulling out the couch she sees one Smartie and one Polo on the carpet, she picks them up and without thinking puts them in her mouth. She reassures herself: they can't possibly have any effect.

The next morning she's regained two pounds and the morning after that, two more - a visit to her grandparents faced her with a stew from which she sneaked the tomatoes and mushrooms but could do nothing about the gravy...

By the end of her first ten days, her weight loss is back to six pounds and Dominic is still sleeping through the night.

Clare's opinion of The NuTron Diet? "Inconclusive - but that's been my fault," she says. "And I have to say I'm preparing some meals I'd never even thought of - everybody loved my chicken livers in soya cream. And the baby makes a lot less mess with rice cakes than Farley's rusks!"

* * *

Anything new - a pair of shoes, a new carpet in the living-room - takes time to get used to and in this respect The NuTron Diet is no different. The thing to remember is that, within a month, it will have become just another part of your daily routine.

The first four weeks are critical and the rules are simple. AVOID EVERYTHING ON YOUR BANNED LIST. EAT ONLY FROM YOUR SAFE LIST. AND IF IN DOUBT - DON'T. Paradoxically, the first sign that the diet is working may be that you feel distinctly unwell - as Clare discovered. But the symptoms rarely last more than a few days. Some people experience no withdrawal symptoms at all. If you're not that fortunate, the message registered on your bathroom scales should cheer you up. Those whose weight problem is retained fluid will find as much as half a stone dropping away over the same few days. The loss may be so considerable that it alarms you - but you have our assurance, it's normal. It may just be advisable to *eat more* - of the foods you're allowed, that is. What is unique about The NuTron Diet is that you CAN EAT AS MUCH AS YOUR APPETITE DEMANDS. If you're concerned that your weight loss is too great, which may be the case if you're having medical treatment, go back to your doctor.

Sticking to the safe list shouldn't be difficult. Indeed, planning meals within it can be enjoyable, as Clare was also beginning to find out; it makes you consider foodstuffs you haven't been in the habit of buying. Staying away from the banned list may be tougher - it depends what's on it. We remember the young woman who reacted only against tomatoes, said "Lovely, I never eat tomatoes," and went happily on her way. If, however, your NuTron Test shows you're intolerant to certain items which are a constituent of other foods, then some effort is required to avoid them.

Clare, for instance, drew a fairly unlucky hand: baker's yeast, which therefore rules out bread and cakes manufactured by the normal process; gluten - which would have ruled out bread if baker's yeast hadn't already done it - but which rules out the wheat, rye, oats and barley that contain it, and foods made from them; whey, which rules out milk and foods made with whey - very common in food processing - or made with milk.

It's understandable, isn't it, that at first Clare felt panic. But food intolerance is a problem you have to meet head on. The NuTron Diet is all or nothing. Choose to ignore that if you want - you won't lose weight.

The seventy or eighty foods left on the average person's safe list after The NuTron Test is hardly a meagre menu. Turn back to page 42 and look at what Clare can choose from - and her list is more restricted than average. But psychologically people resent having restrictions imposed on them and, while very few will have explored anything like the full possibilities of their safe list, they may well decide they're bored by eating from it - though we might add that someone who's suffered from arthritis for twenty years and finds her symptoms disappearing with her extra poundage w̧ probably be happy to stick with her safe list for the rest of her life. However, if after the first four weeks you feel you've got to "break out", you can.

There are two sources for adding variety to your safe list: foods which The NuTron Test have *not* analysed for intolerance, and the foods on the banned list itself. There are several hundred foods which we haven't tested and we suggest you start with some of these. As for the items on the banned list, these are recorded in descending order of intolerant severity. Those bringing up the rear are possibly marginal. It's obvious, therefore, that the re-introduction of foods from the list should start at the bottom. Whether you step into the unknown and try something which The NuTron Test hasn't analysed, or you turn to your banned items, DON'T ADD MORE THAN ONE NEW FOOD AT A TIME. DO EAT THIS FOOD AT LEAST ONCE A DAY FOR THREE OR FOUR DAYS. IF SYMPTOMS SUCH AS A BLINDING HEADACHE, A FEELING OF BLOATING, OR WEIGHT GAIN, OCCUR, THEN STOP - AND ADD THE CULPRIT FOOD TO THE DANGER END OF YOUR LIST.

We also strongly advise you not to drink alcohol, either during the first four weeks or during any subsequent dietary experimentation. Alcohol lends a helping hand in making the intestinal wall permeable - and then gives any food intolerance present a jet-propelled ride around the bloodstream.

If you were intolerant to a food or foods a month ago, how is it that you may not be intolerant now? What you have to realise is that, unknowingly, you've been abusing your immune system *for a lifetime*. Too much sugar and too much carbohydrate - much of which pumps straight out into the bloodstream without the body having a chance to break them down - have made your insulin fire off countless times a day to reduce your

...ntolerance may no longer be an intolerance
...se your immune system is now getting a
... And not having to answer emergency calls to
...to your blood sugar, it's become able to cope with
...things.

Some people may never find that they become tolerant to foods against which they've reacted. Others may find it's safe to go back to foods to which they reacted so badly the test all but blew the haematology analyser off the table. Why different people have such different intolerances is something we don't yet understand. For now, the only way to find out if you can win back your barred foods, and how quickly, is by experiment.

But at the end of the day, it shouldn't really worry you if you're not fortunate. Regard the barred list as peripheral. What matters is the way you look and feel. We predict you'll be so delighted everything else will pale into insignificance.

We've tried to avoid a high moral tone, but from the beginning we've told you there really isn't any cheating with The NuTron Diet - it's all or nothing, certainly to begin with. And that remains true. But there's one measure that you can adopt occasionally which does bend the rules.

Realistically, none of us has total control over what we eat - who knows what's in those dishes we enjoy on holiday, or in those meals out? It's quite possible that food intolerance is lurking, waiting to pounce. Well, you can prevent that happening by asking your GP if he'll prescribe sodium cromoglycate. This drug - specifically developed for the task - coats the wall of the intestine and for a limited period desensitises the mast cells, stopping the chain reaction of food intolerance getting into its stride. It isn't a permanent way of keeping intolerance at bay - it's for that rare infringement only!

* * *

Clare is aware that food intolerance causes hyperactivity and asks us to test her eldest son, Nathan. Hyperactivity is a growing problem now affecting up to twenty percent of children - five times as many boys as girls.

Nathan at seven is a classically hyperactive child. He talks too fast, doesn't listen, can't sit still, always stops whatever he's doing to do whatever someone else is. He has a poor self-image, constantly calls himself stupid, quickly becomes frustrated, sleeps badly and cries at the drop of a hat. He's far from slow, he's aware, but as he never finishes anything, he does badly at school and is now taken by two literacy support teachers. Like all hyperactive children he's exhausting. There are days, Clare says, when his mood swings are so erratic and the tempo of them increases so dramatically that she thinks he'll self-destruct. "On his good days," she adds wryly, "he's like a bluebottle in a jam jar."

Nathan tests intolerant to nineteen foods. Several he never eats, including rabbit - which heads his list - sole and broccoli. But others are chicken, turkey and peas which he likes, just as he likes curry, chilli con carne and pizza but which are now also off the menu because he shares his mother's intolerance to curry powder, chilli pepper and baker's yeast. He also has his mother's intolerance to malt and sugar.

Overall, Clare thinks it's not too bad. Her eldest son is a relatively poor eater who tends to live on cereal and sandwiches. Not having an intolerance to milk and gluten as she does means his cereals are safe, though his favourite, Weetabix, is out because of the malt - and he won't be able to sprinkle his bowl with sugar. As far as bread is concerned, she can switch him to soda bread, which uses bicarbonate of soda rather than baker's yeast as its rising agent.

She stocks up on sugar-free jellies and custard, some fairly expensive sugar-free, yeast-free biscuits - "as insurance or bribes" - and sticks lists of what Nathan can and can't have on the kitchen cupboard, the fridge and the kitchen door.

Clare has taken the baby off a number of the foods she's been feeding him, on the assumption she may have passed her intolerances to him while she was pregnant. The rusks were the first to go, now it's the turn of the Marmite "soldiers" and the Rich Tea Fingers; and Clare gives Dominic soya milk instead of cow's and makes sure he has no added sugar or gravy and that the baby dinners she buys are gluten and egg free.

Now, unfortunately, Dominic develops what Clare's husband, Colin, believes is a bad cold but which she believes are withdrawal symptoms. He doesn't sleep, cries constantly, his eyes, nose and ears run and he has a cough that gradually worsens. Despite her belief, Clare worries that her son may have croup and takes him to the doctor - who can find nothing wrong with him. The next day Dominic's symptoms have totally disappeared - and he's back to sleeping through the night. There's something else: he not only isn't crying, he smiles all the time. Clare can't quite believe it. "Before, he used to cry all the time and I could never make out what he wanted and never knew when to feed him. Now I could set a watch by him - he's gurgling for his breakfast at eight, lunch at twelve, tea at four. It's almost as if I'd been out and got a different baby!"

It's been a fairly traumatic second ten days, but Clare is feeling buoyant, not least because she's had her period without the pre-menstrual tension she's experienced for seventeen years. It's her third period since Dominic was born. "Usually I'm horrible to everyone and I can't help it," she says. "I remember an episode of the TV sitcom 'Roseanne' in which she had PMT and everybody scattered in all directions. I'm afraid it's always been like that in our house, just like most, I suspect. Ask my dad!

"And, usually, I feel tired, bloated and get terrible pains in my back. Since my teens I've intermittently suffered rheumatic pains. Sometimes they affect me so badly I can't bend to pick up one of the children or even drive. And they always get me, every month. But this time - nothing. My period's always arrived like a storm cloud on the horizon and I watch it come towards land, waiting for it to break. This time it caught me by surprise. I felt utterly serene. My husband is the original Doubting Thomas as far as the diet is concerned - but this has got him wavering!"

Clare is also pleased with her experiments with herbal teas, which have very low tannin and are caffeine free: only one has had an adverse effect - cherry rinds - which she supposes is because cherry belongs to the same family as plum and black grape which she's meant to avoid. She can hardly credit the choice: apple and cinnamon, pineapple, blackcurrant leaf, orange and clove... If anything, however, she's even more pleased to have discovered pickles in spirit vinegar rather than malt vinegar. "Unsociable, I know - but I love pickles almost as much as apples."

Her weight loss has remained at six pounds, but she isn't surprised by this. "The six pounds were fluid, the other six I'm sure are fat and will take more time," she says. "But bending over the bath washing my hair I noticed that the triangle of space at the top of my thighs has reappeared - and I haven't seen that for years. And when I walk I'm aware there isn't any wobble in my bottom!"

* * *

What we're about to say now could appear truthfully in any diet book: *processed food is at the lower end of nutritional goodness, can't compete with food that is fresh, and where possible should be replaced in everyone's diet.*

Unless you have a degree in pharmacology, trying to read food labels is like trying to read Sanskrit. Since it became a legal requirement to list ingredients in the order of their predominance, manufacturers have become adept at massaging the truth, sometimes using chemical names instead of ones you'd recognise or listing a thing under a variety of different classifications to disguise the total percentage. And who understands those E numbers? Many customers are unhappy about the use of additives and manufacturers and food chains are cutting down on their use. Our advice on both nutritional and food-avoidance grounds is - stay away from as many processed foods as you can. Taking heed is vital in the context of The NuTron Diet. *If you don't know exactly what's in a food you shouldn't buy it. If it contains an ingredient to which you are intolerant it may prove as dangerous as picking up a hitch-hiker thumbing a lift at the side of the road.*

As far as humanly possible, buy your foods as near to their source as you can get them and as fresh as it's possible to get them. But there's no need to avoid the supermarket, it's a perfectly good supplier of foodstuffs you can trust - particularly around its edges, where the fresh fish counter, the delicatessen, the bakery and the butcher's shop are likely to be. Vary your menu, ensuring it's rich in good protein (which prevents muscle deterioration and wrinkling of the skin) and complex carbohydrates such as whole rice, wholemeal bread and whole-wheat pasta (which are only partly assimilated by the body and therefore produce a much smaller rise in blood sugar than the refined variety). Eat plenty of fresh fruit and vegetables. Keep down your daily intake of sugar, salt and fat, particularly saturated fat. And don't let your tastebuds take precedence over your food intolerances!

At its simplest, The NuTron Diet is the dietary equivalent of Wash and Go. By steering clear of the foods to which the test has shown you to have an intolerance, and by sticking to the foods that it has shown are safe for you, there is nothing else to do in order to lose weight.

The operation does become more difficult if your intolerance involves foods which turn up in disguise in others - gluten, whey, malt, eggs, corn starch and sugar in various combinations are in virtually all packaged foods. If you simply have to buy something in a category where they're common, then you have to turn detective.

The NuTron Test analyses nearly a hundred ingredients. The number of dishes in which that hundred might turn up beggars the imagination. But that isn't important to you as an individual. Your specific list of intolerances narrows the hundred down sharply - and the number of categories of food in which you will have to hunt is manageable.

Try and keep your search to staple items that your banned list has knocked out - and think laterally. If you don't have an intolerance to gluten but, like Clare, you're intolerant to baker's yeast, try soda bread. If you have an intolerance to milk, try soya milk or even coconut milk. If your milk intolerance is only to the lactose, try Lactolite. Soya margarine is as good as any other. If you can't have the Weetabix because you have an intolerance to malt, try Puffed or Shredded Wheat - there's nothing added to the wheat.

We're sure you get the idea. And you'll quickly become adept. You have to stay on the alert, of course, so that you don't let something carrying an intolerance creep under your guard. But once you've done your basic investigation it'll be easy, on a day-to-day basis, to ensure that doesn't happen.

We probably don't have to tell you that the best way of making sure nothing to which you're intolerant gets into your diet - and to ensure the food you eat is the most nutritional - is to prepare and cook it yourself. It's up to you to decide whether you have either the time or the inclination. All we'd add is this: be careful with the incidentals. All your conscientious work will count for nothing if, for example, you have a yeast intolerance and fail to think that the usual gravy granules may contain yeast. Or that, knowing you have an intolerance to sunflower seed/sesame seed/olives, you unthinkingly cook in sunflower oil/sesame oil/olive oil.

A bit of good, old-fashioned common sense will go a long way towards helping you lose weight and retain your weight loss.

* * *

Clare admits to a dark secret. There have been times in the past when she's bundled the children to bed early solely because she wanted to eat a bar of chocolate which she always had hidden in the fridge. "I always felt conscience-stricken, but I couldn't help myself," she says. "I could literally feel my mouth watering thinking

about it. Sometimes the desire
and tear the wrapping off th
irresistible, but I'd never do it w
up because I'd have had to share i

Clare has come to the end of th
days on her NuTron Diet and is tak
had a chocolate craving for more t
feels so strongly that she won't tha
she's able to talk about it - something
not even to her husband.

She wonders to what extent chocolate is at the root of
Nathan's hyperactivity - chocolate contains caffeine,
children are more susceptible to it than adults, and
caffeine is known to have powerful effects, including
inducing mood swings, one of the symptoms of her son's
condition.

She starts Nathan on his diet over the weekend before
half-term, so that she has a clear run of five or six days.
On the Tuesday, Nathan sits down with his mother and
six-year-old sister and plays Monopoly for four-and-a-
half hours. Clare is awestruck - ten minutes is about her
son's usual attention span. The following day he works
on a drawing for school for another four hours. Is it the
diet or is he just trying very hard to please? Any
lingering suspicions Clare might be entertaining on that
score are dispelled a week later when she lets him eat
what he wants at his brother's fourth birthday party
and his tantrums are so explosive everybody is in tears.
"Honestly, it was like watching Dr Jekyll turn into Mr
Hyde," she says.

For the first time in his life Nathan takes a lunchbox
to school - imaginative and flexible as his school's meals
are, they can't accommodate his intolerances. Clare
starts making her own soda bread for his sandwiches -
and discovers Marks and Spencer's Soda Farls. Nathan

with the new arrangement, though he feels deprived in not being able to have a Kit-Kat or a bar like the other children. His mother buys sugar-free milk chocolate from Boots.

And Nathan begins to improve in the classroom - to the extent that he no longer has to attend one of his special classes. His form-teacher tells Clare how helpful he's become, which is something she already knows; in the supermarket Nathan makes a point of reading the labels and telling her what he - and she - can and can't have. "The transformation is beyond belief," Clare says. "When we used to go to the supermarket before, I practically had to lash him to the front of the trolley because he'd run all over the place, shouting, getting into things. I was losing him every five minutes. Now he's angelic.

"Last week a woman was telling off her two children as we went by and I heard her say "I've only got you two and you can't behave. That woman has four and look how good they are." I walked by on air. If only she knew the times I've slunk up to the check-out because Nathan had embarrassed me so much."

As for herself, Clare has lost ten pounds in the month, bringing her weight down to nine stone one pound. "It was twelve pounds until I gave in to temptation and had a pizza," she admits. "I put on the two pounds overnight." What has impressed her is how sensitive her body has become to anything it doesn't like: it lets her know immediately. "We had chicken in yoghurt on Sunday - and yoghurt is obviously something I shouldn't have - and it hit me straight in the back with a pain that climbed into my left shoulder. I understand that the majority of people become less sensitive to their unsafe foods the longer they avoid them, but I don't mind being in the minority. It's a terrific warning system. If I take something to which I'm intolerant, I'm not left in any doubt that I shouldn't have done it!"

While she hopes, at the very least, to re-lose the errant two more pounds ("so I can say I've limbo-danced under the nine-stone barrier") she's already delighted with her transformation, most particularly in her measurements.

On the day before she started The NuTron Diet these were:

Chest:	38in.
Waist:	??
Hips:	38in.
Upper thigh:	21½in.
Lower thigh:	16in.
Calf:	13in.

She refused to measure her waist "because it didn't exist and it disgusted me." At the end of the second ten days, however, after a noticeable reduction, she submitted to the tape. Her waist measurement was 33in.

On the thirtieth day of the diet her measurements were:

Chest:	37in.
Waist:	30in.
Hips:	35in.
Upper thigh:	21in.
Lower thigh:	15in.
Calf:	11in.

That represents an overall loss of fourteen inches - and a drop of one clothes size, from a twelve to a ten. "I'd been squeezing into things that were too small,"

Clare admits. "Now my clothes fit me, and I don't feel like I've been dieting at all. It's difficult to put into words what I feel physically - I feel thinner on the inside. And tauter all over on the outside. And for the first time in my life I haven't got a squidgy jaw line - and I've actually got cheekbones."

And her cynicism about The NuTron Diet? "Believe me, I'm a believer. If you wanted me to go down the street with a billboard round my neck saying 'The End Of The Weight Is Nigh', I would.

"I've even got my wedding ring off for the first time since I was carrying Nathan. I know I set that as a goal at the beginning, but I wasn't really serious about it. But the other night I was taking off my eternity ring and my engagement ring as I do every night and my wedding ring came off with them. It was a very odd moment - one I hadn't experienced for eight years. I felt as if I were being unfaithful. I got into bed but then got out and put my eternity and engagement rings back on. I didn't feel I belonged to anybody!"

Between the end of her first month's NuTron Diet and publication of this book - a period of three months - Clare lost another five pounds, bringing her weight to eight stone ten. Her measurements: chest (36 ½in), waist (27in), hips (34in), upper thigh (20½in), lower thigh (14½in) and calf (11in), represent a total loss of 20½ inches from the beginning of the diet.

FROM GENES TO JEANS

Sex is the engine of life. Sex is the most powerful desire in almost every living thing. The healthiest members of every species breed the healthiest offspring. And while for humans good sex isn't exclusively enjoyed by the healthy, being healthy undoubtedly leads to good sex.

It's just as certain that being overweight leads to less enjoyable sex. And being overweight, as we've told you time and again, is likely to be the result of food intolerance. Food intolerance really is the enemy in our midst. If it were responsible only for the misery caused to so many people who are overweight, that would be bad enough. But it spreads its malign influence into almost all areas and these include those associated with sex, both recreational and procreational.

The notion that a woman says no because she has a headache may be a music-hall joke, but it's only a joke because it's based on an observed fact. The mechanism that makes people want to have sexual intercourse involves a complex and delicate interplay of body chemistry and cerebral motivation. The pain of a headache - worse, a migraine - knocks out the mechanism. The libido is just as discouraged by depression, anxiety, mental exhaustion, lack of energy and a wide variety of minor symptoms that both males and females suffer - ALL OF WHICH CAN BE BROUGHT ON BY FOOD INTOLERANCE.

Women pay a far higher price then men for food

intolerance because of their reproductive function: ten million in the UK alone suffer pre-menstrual tension and many, many more are at the mercy of irregular, painful or heavy periods, with the monthly unpleasantness of abdominal bloating, breast tenderness, fluid accumulation - and temporary weight gains that may be half a stone or more. Cystitis, an inflammation of the bladder which at its mildest induces a slight burning when passing water but which can be so painful and debilitating that it leaves women in a constant state of embarrassment and worry, can also make intercourse impossible.

Most doctors treat cystitis with antibiotics. No-one would deny that antibiotics have saved countless lives since their introduction into medicine in the 1940s and there are times, unquestionably, when they're needed. But antibiotics have been prescribed too frequently, often when simple alternative measures would have been just as effective, and their use has the harmful side-effect of stripping valuable organisms from the bowel - which gives candida the freedom to play havoc.

Millions of organisms friendly to their host coat the wall of the healthy intestine and exercise "crowd control" over candida. Of these, the lactobacilli, the most prolific and beneficial, produce biotin, part of the vitamin B complex, and other substances. Once antibiotics kill off some of the bacilli, candida colonises and, moreover, gets a grip on the intestine wall - where it probably assists food intolerances to prise open the mast cells.

The body's immune system tries to keep the candida at bay, but may be overwhelmed by the multiplying organisms. If the battleground is the vagina, the likelihood is that the irritant white curd-like discharge of thrush will make an appearance. A woman who's experienced heavy or painful periods from the onset of menstruation in her teens almost certainly was treated with antibiotics in her childhood; candida could well have started invading her womb and ovaries from puberty.

Once, removing children's tonsils was the standard treatment for tonsillitis, something that was usually unnecessary and made as much sense as ripping a fire alarm off the wall. Nowadays, tonsillitis is more likely to be treated with antibiotics - less brutal, but bringing with it the problem that the child's intestinal lactobacilli are often stripped away, inducing candidiasis. That is also the case with a common childhood ailment these days, glue ear, which causes hearing difficulties and makes children slow to learn to speak and, often, to display behavioural difficulties. Every year in this country, sixty thousand three and four-year-olds undergo an operation to have grommets inserted in their ears as a result of glue ear, at a cost to the NHS of £30 million. It's a sobering thought that there is now some evidence that grommets can lead to long-term hearing loss. Perhaps it's just as sobering to think that many of these children might not have needed to enter hospital at all, had their mothers, while pregnant, known that there were foods they should avoid - and by avoiding them they would decrease the likelihood of the foetus in their womb being predisposed to the condition.

That a woman who smokes during pregnancy is storing up for her unborn infant a life-time of distress is now universally accepted and the vast majority of pregnant women don't smoke. *Universal recognition that food intolerance could be an even greater danger - greater, not least, in its insidiousness, working as it does under cover of a mother's belief that what she's eating is benefiting her and her baby - would be the biggest leap forward there's ever been in pre-natal care.*

As an aside - but a very important aside - we'd make the point that both the Pill and Hormone Replacement Therapy have much the same effect as antibiotics in that they promote the growth of candida. Many women on the Pill are known to be at increased risk of developing thrush. The Pill also leads to deficiencies in essential nutrients, especially zinc, vitamin C, vitamin B6 and other B vitamins. This makes the immune system less efficient - leaving the body less capable of resisting a candida invasion. Should a woman come off the Pill to start a family and immediately succeed in becoming pregnant, she will lose more nutrients from her depleted store. The risk could be a difficult pregnancy or a problem labour.

While HRT may help to prevent brittle bone disease after the menopause, it doesn't vary the blood levels in the way it occurs in the natural state and candidiasis is more likely to develop. It's advisable for a woman to sort out her food intolerances before the menopause, which will allow the change to take place more smoothly. In a healthy woman, the amount of oestrogen put out by the ovaries gradually wanes and, eventually, virtually stops - but it continues in small amounts over many years, still being produced by the adrenal glands. There is some evidence that food intolerance suppresses the natural output or causes its sudden demise.

In terms of weight gain and other consequences of food intolerances, men pay the same price as women, but a woman's physiology makes her especially vulnerable. Cystitis and thrush are conditions that can make her fear having sex. PMT subjects her to mood swings that are unpredictable, uncontrollable and, perhaps, violent. Some women suffer symptoms - which include clumsiness, low self-esteem, a tendency to say the wrong thing or to be ultra-sensitive about what's said - that last from ovulation to the end of their period. That gives a one-week window for a happy sex life - if, that is, an attack of cystitis or thrush doesn't crop up and assuming that PMT hasn't made any kind of relationship impossible.

What is startling is that so much human unhappiness is caused by something so apparently trivial as food intolerance - something which can now be pin-pointed and put to rights by The NuTron Diet.

* * *

Healthy people, generally speaking, have healthy babies. Why other people have babies that are unhealthy, or lose babies during pregnancy, or even fail to conceive, are questions that may have complex and difficult answers. The simple answer in many cases is food intolerance.

A child is conceived when male sperm and female egg unite to form a single cell that contains an equal number of genes from each parent. These genes are arranged along twenty-three pairs of chromosomes - the DNA chains that will carry the genetic code in every cell of the child's body - one of each pair contributed by each parent. Genes are the building blocks of heredity. In their new - and unique - combination they will determine whether the child is male or female and what its characteristics will be.

Well, and good. But what effect does the nutritional health of the parents play?

Any couple wanting a child have the responsibility of giving it the best start in life they can. Ensuring that their own bodies are healthy before their child's conception should be their very first step.

A failure to conceive may have physical causes. If that isn't the case, the nutrient state of either partner is likely to be responsible. Quite often women don't become pregnant because of a simple nutrient deficiency (notably zinc); many more, we believe, fail because their blood has been polluted by toxins spilled from damaged white blood cells - a situation caused by food intolerance.

The inability to have children causes a great deal of misery and is responsible for the break-down of innumerable relationships. Some couples never ascertain the underlying cause. Some blame each other. Some, determined to become parents at any cost, subject themselves to examination that can be humiliating and almost certainly expensive.

One woman who'd spent £10,000 in Harley Street for unsuccessful treatment over several years, came to us in desperation. Her NuTron Test showed that she reacted against red wine, chocolate, cheese, tea and coffee. She gave them all up. And - as well as losing a lot of weight - a year later she conceived. Hers is not an isolated case.

Conception should only occur when the body is able to support it, but there's a sliding scale in such matters. Sometimes the body allows conception, then reassesses the situation and changes its mind. The result can be a miscarriage. One woman in five experiences bleeding in the first three months of pregnancy, which indicates a risk factor. Not all end in miscarriage but, unfortunately, far too many do. When one takes account of the women who miscarry so early that they haven't even been aware of their conception the enormity of the problem begins to come into focus.

A body that's not at ease with its pregnancy can dysfunction in other ways: ectopic pregnancy (in which the fertilised egg becomes embedded in the wall of a

Fallopian tube instead of in the uterus) is common; and pre-eclampsia (pregnancy-induced hypertension), which in rare cases can kill mother or child or both. Even if a pregnancy that the body ought not to have allowed goes full term, the consequences can be tragic: the birth of a child with Down's Syndrome, perhaps, or spina bifida.

Thanks to advances in medical technology and pre-natal diagnosis there is a range of screening tests that doctors can offer expectant mothers: ultrasound, amniocentesis and chorionic villus sampling, the MSAFP or AFP test, and others. Sadly, abnormalities are becoming all too common.

It would be foolish and immoral to claim that The NuTron Test can guarantee success for every childless couple, or that every pregnant woman who identified and eliminated her food intolerances would never have to endure a screening procedure that might face her with the agonising decision of termination. *What we do say is that The NuTron Diet can go a long way towards helping eliminate many problems associated with childbirth - a quick, simple and comparatively inexpensive way of fulfilling so many hopes and expectations.*

* * *

If you were to pick up any current guidebook on dieting in pregnancy - and hadn't read a word that we've written about food intolerance - you would think the advice given by them is highly sensible.

There are, you would read, four main food groups: starchy foods (complex carbohydrates) which include wholemeal bread, breakfast cereals, dried fruit and jacket potatoes (providing protein, fibre, vitamins, minerals and energy); dairy produce, including milk, cheese, yoghurt (calcium, protein, vitamin A, zinc, iodine, magnesium); meat and fish, including alternatives - eggs, nuts, beans (protein, vitamins A and B, fibre - in nuts and beans - iron, zinc); and fruits and vegetables (vitamins A, C, folic acid, fibre, potassium and iron). Popularly, the advice would be that an expectant mother should have four or more servings daily from group one, four from group two, three from group three and four from group four - from which group one serving should be of dark yellow or green leafy vegetables and one serving from citrus fruits or tomatoes. Small amounts of sugary food and drinks, you would be told, are allowed in moderation.

Millions of women follow this advice in good faith. On the face of it, such advice couldn't be better. But enter food intolerance into the equation - and the highly nutritional diet becomes a time-bomb.

The last of Clare Hickman's four pregnancies came to the end of its term more than six months before she took a NuTron Test and discovered what her intolerances were (refresh your memory by having another look at pages 41-42). Had she known earlier, she would NOT have eaten:

• Wholemeal bread (intolerant to gluten, baker's yeast, malt)

• Weetabix/Shredded Wheat and milk (intolerant to gluten, whey) sprinkled with extra bran (gluten)

• Cheese - her lunch usually consisted of various varieties with butter (whey) and cream crackers (gluten, yeast, malt extract), followed by a yoghurt (candida reaction to sugar). She also developed an addiction to Dairylea cheese "triangles" which she nibbled throughout the day

• Egg and tomato salad (intolerant to egg white and tomato) - her lunch alternative

Add to this list the gravy (yeast, wheat flour) that invariably accompanied the evening meal she prepared, the hot chocolate (candida reaction) she constantly drank and the ginger beer (brewer's yeast) which became a daily item after she'd read that ginger stopped morning sickness, and you can see that both the core and the periphery of Clare's diet were doing her as much harm as good.

Her weight gain was almost double the recommended figure - she went from nine stone to twelve. "And I was sick all the time," she says. "I'd been sick with the other three, but nothing like the last. I think I thought it was a normal progression. Now I'm convinced my food intolerances had built up to the point where they were spilling over."

The plain fact is, any dietary advice that doesn't take account of individual food intolerances - and until now none has been able to - is quite useless. No-one would make jackets, skirts and trousers all in one size and assume they'd fit everybody. So it is with diets. YOUR diet has to be tailored to fit YOU. If it's not, then it's as futile as...well, calorie counting.

It's no wonder, is it, that so many seemingly healthy women like Clare who eat responsibly during pregnancy, avoid alcohol and cigarettes, and religiously follow their exercise programmes, still experience symptoms that include fatigue, irritability, headaches, painful joints and muscles - and that ever-present feeling of sickness.

Birth itself should be an uncomplicated business but, again, many women experience difficulties, going into labour early or late, struggling to produce quite small babies, having to be delivered by caesarean section, subsequently having problems with breast feeding, falling victim to post-natal depression.

Food intolerance undermines the body's democratic rule. It encourages candida to outbreaks of anarchy almost anywhere in the body. It triggers hypoglycaemia which leads to swings in blood sugar. It causes fluid to leak into muscles and tissue. It affects the immune system. What chance does it have of *not* affecting the baby in the womb and at the breast?

This cycle, you'll agree, is depressing, and those working in the nutritional field over many years have only been able to wring their hands, even while gathering more and more evidence. A study in New Zealand, for instance, found that colic was worst in babies whose mothers ate eggs, fish, milk, chocolate and nuts, which are commonly implicated as food intolerances, but also as food allergies in the way immunologists define the term. Another study in the Isle of Wight took lactating mothers off a series of commonly allergenic foods and found that "hereditary" illnesses (mainly asthma and eczema) in one-year-old babies dropped from 40% to 13%.

The problem with these and many other studies was that there was no specific and accurate way of identifying individual food reactions. But now there's The NuTron Test which does - *the breakthrough that should change pregnancy and motherhood from the frequently distressing experience it has been into the joyful one it should be.*

* * *

Pregnancy is a time when even a woman who's an ardent weight watcher tends to ease up on herself. Pregnant women, after all, are supposed to gain weight.

This is true. The question is: how much? The answer, taking account of the weight of the baby, the amniotic fluid and placenta, the increase in the womb and in the breasts ready for feeding - and the extra blood for the whole process - should be twenty or twenty-five pounds at full term.

But many women far exceed this kind of weight gain and, indeed, never return to their pre-pregnancy weight. Anyone who's read this book this far already knows why. Candida may be on the march, multiplying furiously in the bowel and inducing carbohydrate craving that the woman indulges. Her diet of sugary concoctions and refined carbohydrates turn her bloodstream into a kind of Piña Colada in which the candida feeds to its heart's content, almost invariably making an appearance in the area of the vagina where the sugar around the uterus sustains the foetus. Meanwhile, the insulin is snatching away what sugar it can and pushing it out as fat, to keep the blood sugar level normal. And the capillaries, made permeable by the toxic fallout from the damaged neutrophils, are leaking fluid all over the place.

All of this is caused by the food intolerance that allowed the undigested food particles, and the candida, through the gut wall in the first place - what is quite simply called "The Leaking Gut Syndrome".

Once it was thought that the placenta acted like a kind of Thames Barrier against toxic substances crossing over from the mother's bloodstream to the foetus. The thalidomide tragedy of the early 1960s showed how very wrong that was - and there's substantial evidence that alcohol, drugs and carbon monoxide and nicotine from cigarette smoke also pass through the placenta, with harmful results including dependency.

We would add food intolerance to this small but ugly list. Just as surely as an expectant mother's smoking or drinking affects her unborn child, so do her food intolerances - both, after all, share the same bloodstream.

It means that a food intolerance that causes discomfort (such as a headache) to a mother can do the same thing to her baby - the baby may be kicking experimentally but it may equally be in distress. It means that a mother's intolerances to specific foods are likely to be transferred so that when her baby is born it, too, will suffer from them. That is also true of a number of medical conditions. Yet by eliminating her food intolerances, a woman can not only eradicate such a condition in herself - she'll help prevent it exhibiting itself in the baby in her womb.

The implications for any atopic family - that is, one which has a history of a specific illness or condition that is passed from generation to generation - are enormous.

And - if we might appeal to the expectant mother's vanity - she'll pass the jeans test within weeks of having her baby. Is there a woman in the country who hasn't judged whether she's got back her figure by trying to get into her pre-pregnancy jeans? And, very probably, been reduced to tears because she's failed? The NuTron Test and the individual diet which results from it are the Dynamic Duo that will come to her rescue!

DON'T TAKE OUR WORD FOR IT!

People come in all shapes and sizes. Some are merely overweight, others have a medical condition to contend with as well. Some have stones to lose, other pounds. The NuTron Diet can help them all, as these case histories show - *but only if the rules are obeyed.*

* * *

Eleanor Verity. Age: 55. Height: 5ft 1in. Weight before The NuTron Diet: 16st 3lbs. Office Manager .
"Overweight runs in my family and I've always been on diets. In 1971 I got down to ten stone and was one of a slimming magazine's slimming champions of the year, but it took me a year and I had to starve myself. Not long after that my first husband died and I stopped taking care about what I was eating - I suppose eating was some kind of compensation. During the last twenty years I'd tried every kind of diet and got off half a stone at different times, but it always came back and I'd stayed around fourteen-fifteen stone.

In February 1992 I began to feel a pain in my breast and thought it was a heart problem. When I went to the doctor he said it was inflammation of the muscles of the chest wall though he didn't say exactly what it was. By the November I was very ill. The pain had become excruciating and had spread to my arms, legs and joints. At night I had to support my left leg with one pillow and my left arm with another, I couldn't get out of bed or drive the car and I needed help to get dressed or have a bath. I was in tears the whole time. In January 1993 I was seen by a specialist, underwent a lot of tests and was told that what I had was polymyositis, a disease that's fairly rare and causes inflammation of the muscles and joints - as if I didn't know. I was told it would take up to six years for the disease to get out of my system and I'd have to live with it.

For fifteen years I'd been visiting officer for a district council processing housing benefit claims but in May 1993 I had to take early retirement because of the state of my health. It was a worrying time. My second husband Paul is a gardener and we have a tied cottage, but his wage is fairly low and while I had a pension and invalidity benefit I wasn't sure we could manage with a daughter just going to college.

Paul wears headphones while he's gardening and he was listening to Radio Sussex when Ian [Stoakes] was interviewed about the blood test and he said it sounded like a really good idea - but I was actually too ill to care. Then by one of those strokes of good luck I was introduced to Ian - at a bring-and-buy sale. I had good days and bad days and this was one of my good days, so I'd gone to run my stall, though, of course, I had to sit on a chair.

I was taking steroids and I'd shot up to sixteen stone three pounds and hated the look of myself, fenders at the back and a veranda at the front. I couldn't look in the mirror. Ian offered to test me and I said yes, but I honestly didn't think it would do any good.

When I got the results I didn't look at the green side, just the red and all the things I'd lose: milk and grains (except rice), cheese, rhubarb and brussels sprouts which I love, tomatoes, coffee, cabbage, corn. Still, I decided to go through with it. My daughter took me shopping and we spent three hours in the supermarket reading every packet and every tin. I was horrified because corn starch seemed to be in everything. Even now I'd kill for a corn-on-the-cob. But I've grown to like rice cakes - after a bit of shopping round I'd recommend the sesame seed variety to anybody - and rice pudding made with soya cream is delicious.

In the first ten days I lost six pounds, seven pounds in the next ten. By then I was feeling so much better I was even driving the car, though only short distances. Within two months I'd dropped twenty-three pounds and was feeling so good I was offered a job as office manager. Anybody seeing me running up and down the stairs all day would never guess that a while ago I couldn't even get upstairs. And my eczema has virtually disappeared. As a child I suffered very badly from that, even having to wear splints in bed at night so as not to scratch myself, and I once ended up in hospital having temporarily lost my sight when the eczema got under my eyelids and I couldn't stop rubbing them. The condition improved markedly with the birth of my children but it was always with me, sometimes badly. Now it's barely detectable at the base of my fingers.

What I find remarkable is that I've lost any weight at all because I'm still on steroids, though they're much reduced and I expect to be finished with them soon. I still get the odd achey day but it's nothing compared to what I was suffering. I'm ashamed to admit that there was one week when I felt miserable, said blow the diet, as every overweight person does, ate everything I shouldn't quite deliberately and put on six pounds in three days - and felt so awful I had to go to the physiotherapist with a problem with my neck. I won't be doing that again!

I still can't believe how lucky I am. The diet has given me a new lease of life. At fifty-five I thought I'd never work again and I'd be stuck at home, which I hate. And being in the place where other people are being helped is giving me terrific satisfaction. People ring up and say: "Will it really work?" And I tell them about me - and that swings it for them."

* * *

Doctor Raj Dhumali, MBBS, MS, FRCS. Age: 40. Height: 5ft 9in. Weight before The NuTron Diet: 12st 7lbs. A former heart surgeon he's spent three years re-training as a GP and is currently looking for a practice.

"For the last five years I've been into Chinese kick boxing and have reached black belt level. I took it up because working as a heart surgeon at St George's, Tooting, and then Broadgreen Hospital, Liverpool, had made me fat and flabby. Paradoxically there I was, saving other people's lives, but while my brain was functioning I was standing around in the theatre all day, or else eating unhealthy cheese sandwiches like everybody else and breathing in cigarette smoke - the other doctors all smoked like hell. I think I was killing myself.

I was drawn to martial arts because of the discipline - it's mental as well as physical and there's a goal. Squash, circuit training, jogging all seem pretty pointless to me. And it's much harder than any of them - you're well protected but it's a full-contact sport and you have to put in at least two three-hour sessions a week and better three or four.

I started off at nearly fourteen stone and came back to

twelve-and-a-half, but that was still half a stone above my ideal weight. I couldn't shift it no matter how strenuously I trained so I reduced my calorie intake to 1,500 a day for three months. I had to grit my teeth I can tell you - it helped that I was doing a sponsored weight loss for Romania. But I made no inroads into that half stone.

When I was asked to take part in the placebo cross-over trial I was sceptical about a diet based on eliminating food intolerances - initially that is. I still believed that calorie reduction should work, which goes to show that you can specialise in one area of medicine and lose complete touch with everything else. I just thought like every other member of the public.

When I heard the food intolerance theory of overweight - particularly what it had to say about fluid retention - it made absolute sense to me and I thought: why the hell didn't I think of this before? I hadn't thought it through, though I already knew I was hyper-allergic to lentils and certain spices.

It was no surprise that lentils came up on my list of intolerances. Others were coffee, milk, mackerel, egg white, brewer's yeast, malt - and curry powder. I was less than pleased with these last three because I enjoy a whisky in the evening and a few lagers at the weekend and, of course, curries are a part of my heritage. But I kept to the diet for the length of the trial. And quite magically my weight dropped to twelve stone.

I have to say that my weight has gone back up to thirteen stone in recent weeks, but that's because I've been sitting around studying for exams and not exercising - and because, as a matter of choice, I haven't kept to the diet. I enjoy my whisky and my lager just as I enjoy my lentils, spices and curries and I'm not prepared to give any of them up. I believe in the quality of my life above my weight and if the price is a mild itch or a bit of bloating, then that's the way it is. I do think the concept of food intolerance has an important part to play in slimming, especially for those who need to lose weight seriously. For my part, I'm glad to know the diet's there - when I need to lose weight for a competition I now know I can do it."

* * *

Christine Haign. Age: 46. Height: 5ft 3in. Weight before The NuTron Diet: 13st. Private school teacher and former Salvation Army Officer.

"Bingeing was my problem. I would eat a decent evening meal - and then go out to the kitchen and have four slices of bread and jam. If I made sandwiches for one of the children it would be an excuse to make some for myself. The bingeing varied with my mood and my cycle but it had reached a point where I was out of control.

I used to weigh ten-and-a-half stone but that had gradually increased and in the last two years I hadn't fluctuated by more than about half a stone. I'd been to Weight Watchers, and tried other diets. Sometimes I calorie counted, even cutting down to 1,000 a day, sometimes not. I was inconsistent. Whatever I did it didn't last. Foodwise, I was never satisfied - the craving never went and I was embarrassed and depressed about it. My weight was making me very unfit - I was getting very short of breath. It didn't help that the chronic rheumatism that I'd had for twenty years was getting worse in my hips and legs. I hadn't had time off work but it was costing me a lot to keep going.

Eventually I went to the doctor who rather suggested that the problem was in my mind and he gave me water tablets that were no help at all. I just felt despair. I knew my problem was physical, not mental - I'd had a breakdown and was ill in 1979-80 so I knew what that was like and this wasn't like that at all. I knew I had a problem that is fairly common with women, but I couldn't go back to the doctor who hadn't treated me like an individual, just another middle-aged woman.

I was willing to try anything by the time my husband Philip mentioned taking a blood test for food intolerance. I'd cut out some things in the past which had given some relief from the rheumatism and I knew that special diets were of benefit in certain health situations.

I tested intolerantly to eighteen items that included a few things I don't eat but which also included baker's yeast and gluten, which meant goodbye to bread, and things like mushroom, curry, coffee and black pepper.

The first two or three days were very difficult. I had terrible headaches and craved and craved. Then everything settled down and I began to feel better within two weeks; within four weeks I'd lost nine pounds and by the time we went on holiday two weeks later - armed with soya milk and rice cakes - I was feeling really good. But we were away three weeks, the stuff I brought ran out, the local bread was too good to resist, I got careless - and I came home having put on nine pounds, with swollen hands and face, my joints seized up and feeling absolutely dreadful. It took me a month to get back to where I was.

In the beginning I found it difficult to have food around me that I wasn't allowed and for a while the family had to go without bread, but I'm over that now. And it's very rare now that I look at any food and think "I can't have that", where before almost everything was a temptation. I don't bother cooking special things because with a full-time job it's difficult. Just as importantly, though, I don't feel the need to replace the things I can't have - I just don't feel deprived.

I've lost nearly two stone, but, if anything, I'm more grateful for the improvement in my health than in my weight loss though people remark on that. There hasn't been much effect on my frozen left shoulder, but the change everywhere else has been remarkable. I'm moving comfortably and freely again and I haven't been this supple since I was twenty-six. I don't flag like I used to. And everyone says I look perkier."

***

*Beryl Waters. Age: 63. Height: 5ft. Weight before
The NuTron Diet: 12st. 7lbs. Owns a grocery/off-
licence with her husband and son.*

"For twenty years I attended slimming clubs, for twelve years I was on tablets for water retention, ever since I can remember I religiously ate three slices of wholemeal bread and drank a pint of skimmed milk every day - and it was all a waste of time.

I was at the slimming club where the first experiment was carried out with this blood test diet and I jumped at the chance of being one of the volunteers. Well, jumped is an exaggeration. When you've got bad arthritis in both knees you don't jump much. But I lost eight pounds in ten days or something like that. I'd never achieved anything like that before. Keith my husband was thrilled but furious: "You've gone all these years and the doctor never suggested anything like that," he said.

I have a chair at the back of the shop. But I can be on my feet all day and things were getting so I couldn't do it. I couldn't get up or down kerb edges without holding on to things. I'd got so as I was frightened to go into town and I'd been to the doctor to see about one new knee joint, and been to see the specialist. When I told the doctor about the blood test he put his arm around my shoulder and said: "Don't pin your hopes on it, love."

Whether I did or I didn't, it worked. I'm now under eleven stone and I don't go to the slimming club. I'm doing it all by myself. I haven't had to worry about a new knee joint, either, the arthritis is so much better. Before, I couldn't use the steps in the shop and I couldn't reach up to things which I can do now. And I can get hold of things - before my fingers were crippled with the arthritis. People coming into the shop are amazed at how I look. Sometimes I can't believe it myself.

I go into town all the time now. I'm not going to say I can walk all round town, and I do get a taxi back, but I'm mobile again. I can go up and down stairs, too - one step at a time, but without any problem. Yet people used to gather to watch me get off kerbs. I now look at women with big thick legs and I think how easily they could change the way they look if only they knew. No-one needs to be misshapen, and that's what water does to you. That's why I started to have my clothes made, I couldn't buy anything. Now I can. But I still have some of my clothes made - they're smarter.

I've been tested twice - the first test only had thirty items on it. But the second test didn't make much of a difference really. The first one showed I was intolerant to gluten, milk, tea and coffee and the yeasts. The second only added other minor things and things we don't have like crab. We like plain English foods, not curries and things like that. I can have meat and veg and that's what we like. Cutting out coffee and the bread and milk were the main things.

I don't knock slimming clubs. They do good and it's not their fault they don't know about the blood test.

But that doctor. He knew nothing about water retention. I'll never forget him putting his arm around me and saying "Don't pin your hopes on it, love.' He's retired now."

* * *

Janet Jobbins. Age: 28. Height: 5ft 2in. Weight before The NuTron Diet: 14st.7lbs. Credit controller in PR and sports sponsorship company.

"I am a psychologically bad eater. I won't eat fruit or vegetables that make a crunching noise or have a fleshy texture - apples, cucumber, even lettuce. I love orange juice but I couldn't bear to eat an orange because of the fleshy texture. Anything that crunches or has a "feel" in my mouth makes me heave. I've been like it ever since I was tiny - I have a memory from about the age of two of being made by my mother to sit where I was until I finished my broad beans and I wouldn't no matter what she did. I'm so bad with food that my husband David, who's a restaurant manager, won't take me out for a meal.

When I was tested I proved intolerant to quite a lot of things including fish and cheese that I don't touch - fish to which I'm allergic and can't eat, though I wouldn't mind, and cheese, which I'll have on top of shepherd's pie or something like that but which I couldn't eat on its own. The main ones as far as I was concerned were chicken, rice, and sugar, which meant no cakes or syrup on pancakes which I love. In fact, the diet forbade all the things I live on.

I've been on all sorts of diets, micro diets, liquid diets. I haven't so much calorie counted as tried to cut down. But in the last five years I've stayed much the same weight, unable to get any off but at least not putting it on.

It was a terrible shock having to do without the things I like but I did it, living mostly on spaghetti bolognaise, and in the first ten days the weight fell off. I lost ten-and-a-half pounds. But then I went back to eating normal things - I just found doing without the few things I am able to eat impossible day in and day out.

I admit I could have tried harder. I wasn't intolerant to gluten or milk and didn't have a candida reaction. But, again, so many things have a texture I can't stand - I could eat pizza, though I'm not fond of it, but it's almost impossible to get one without something on top that I have to scrape off. And it's a matter of lifestyle. I work full-time and when I get in I'm tired, I don't want to cook and I want to grab the first thing in the fridge. I also have to put Timothy to bed. He's twenty-two months now and a big lad - thirty pounds. He was born three months early and weighed three pounds, ten ounces. At least I'm making sure he eats his vegetables - I'm determined he won't grow up like me.

It's a couple of months since I gave up the diet and I haven't put any weight back on. But that's because I've been quite ill - I've had lockjaw because of a wisdom tooth. I'm quite sure the weight will come back now I'm better.

I'd love to be eight stone. I work in an office with twenty-eight girls and they all seem to be a size ten. We had the company photograph taken recently and I'm the blob in the middle. But you have to make choices and I've made mine, even if I am being a fool to myself.

* * *

THE NUTRON DIET

Julia Nelson. Age: 62. Height: 5ft 4in. Weight before
The NuTron Diet: 11st.
Church of England schools officer.

"I went into hospital for a dual operation on an arthritic knee - a cartilage and a sebaceous cyst - and came out, not with the cure I'd hoped for, but with a problem I was told I'd have to live with for the rest of my life. If that's the case, I thought, I ought to lose half a stone to take the strain off my knee, and that's why I went to the surgery - where I learnt about the new diet.

I have to say I was sceptical at first and perhaps more so when I got my list of things to which I was intolerant. I could somehow accept the baker's yeast and the gluten, though that rather said goodbye to bread, biscuits, pastries and cakes. But I also had salmon and coconut on my list and I thought that was ridiculous. Anyway, I stuck to what it was safe for me to eat - and enjoyed things I hadn't touched before like baked potatoes and roast parsnips, as well as things I didn't eat though I loved, like sautéed mushrooms, because I thought they were bad for me. And I lost thirteen pounds, a loss I've maintained. I even eat chocolate.

In my thirties and forties I used to go on a diet and lose half a stone without too much difficulty. It gets very hard or even impossible when you're older. Three years ago I went on a very strict diet using my calorie counting tables and reduced my intake to 1,200 calories a day. And I got absolutely nowhere. To have lost thirteen pounds in a month was absolutely amazing.

Being the person I am I still didn't believe the business of the coconut and the salmon so I tried a curry with coconut - and I went bananas, if I can put it like that. The most frightful headache and light-headedness. On another occasion I tried salmon steaks and the next morning I'd put on three or four pounds. It's all very

86

strange and I don't understand it at all, but now I'm a confirmed believer. My daughter suffers from bad migraines and I'm trying to persuade her to have the test.

As the weather's got colder I've got out outfits I haven't been able to get into for years and people keep complimenting me on how I look. And I have to say I feel fantastic. As for the arthritis, it's got a good deal better, instead of being the on-going process of deterioration I was told to expect. We went on holiday to Jordan this year and at the Valley of Tombs in Petra I was one of only six people who climbed the seven hundred steps to the top. I felt so good I just did it."

* * *

Dave Williams. Age: 48. Height: 5ft 10 ¹/₂ in.
Weight before The NuTron Diet: 25st. 7lbs.
Social Club Manager.

"I went to the surgery with an abscess on my nose - and came out having agreed to go on this new diet. I'd been on diets before - doctor's diets, egg diets, grapefruit diets. One time I broke my ankle and the hospital put me on something so strict it was ridiculous and I lost a stone. And I'd been to Weight Watchers - lost thirty-seven pounds over ten weeks doing the old calorie counting, but I was hungry all the time and really depressed.

My weight bothers other people, but it's never bothered me. I was always big. Weighed sixteen stone when I left school. Used to do power lifting which kept me down to twenty-one or twenty-two stone, but I'd stopped that and the weight had crept up to twenty-five. Twenty-five stone's a bit much for anybody and I thought, well, give this new diet a go.

I do like my food. Took me back a bit when I saw the things I couldn't have - knocked out bread, milk, tea, beef, tomatoes and mushrooms and some other things like strawberries and bananas. Still, I could eat as much as I liked of anything else. And I could still have a drink - I have anywhere from six to twelve bottles of Pils a night. You have to drink to be sociable in my job.

I had my doubts the diet could work - I mean, it wasn't like any other diet I'd ever heard of. But it did - two-and-a-half stone dropped off me in three weeks. Mind, I had terrible withdrawal symptoms the first week. Woke up one night shivering and cold and had to come down for a slice of bread and butter. Felt perfectly all right in ten minutes but I'd put on four pounds next day.

I really missed the beef, but I can have lamb, pork, chicken, fish, jacket potatoes, whatever veg I want. I don't feel restricted, I don't feel the need to cheat and I haven't bothered to find any substitutes. You can't complain about a diet that lets you eat a cooked breakfast - on my day off me and the wife go to a Little Chef and I regularly have two eggs, bacon, beans, sausages, the lot, except the fried bread. And the weight's still going down - seven-and-a-half stone in six months. I haven't been under twenty stone in more than twenty years. I'm thinking now I might even get back to sixteen stone.

I've never had any problems being overweight but I realise now how much better I feel. I'd had an ulcer for twenty years and was taking Tagamet daily, but I've stopped that now. I've even started doing a bit of training. The darts season's just started and I'm going into pubs I haven't been into since last season and everybody notices. Some people don't recognise me. The only drawback is the clothes - I've gone down four sizes. My waist was fifty inches and that's now forty. I've lost two inches off my neck and six off my chest. We sorted out the wardrobe the other day and got shot of sixteen pairs of trousers, three jackets and I don't know how many shirts. I've the confidence I'll not be needing them."

* * *

Christine Sellars. Age: 14. Height: 5ft. 4in.
Weight before The NuTron Diet: 14st 2lbs.
Her story is told by her mother Lyn, an estate agent.

"I've always felt guilty about Christine. She was conceived when my husband and I were on a weekend holiday in Amsterdam, although I didn't know that until eight weeks later. In the meantime I puffed my duty free cigarettes, and the allowance my husband, a non-smoker, brought back. Once I knew I was pregnant, I stopped smoking and have never gone back to it. But it's always been in the back of my mind that in those first vital weeks my smoking starved Christine of oxygen in my womb.

Right from birth she cried a lot, had colic, reacted badly to several milks until we found one that she seemed able to take. If there was anything going round when she was a child she got it: tonsillitis, sore throats, ear infections. She reacted very badly to her first whooping cough jab and I was advised not to let her have the other two, but whenever she had a cough I spent days in a constant state of worry. She always had the sniffles.

Until she was about eleven her weight was normal. Even when she started putting on weight I was pleased because for a year or two she seemed much more like other girls her age. I know she ate too much junk food, too many sweets, drank too many Cokes - and wouldn't sit down to a proper meal unless I practically stood over her with a gun to her head. But that's what youngsters are like today and I thought the weight she was carrying was only puppy fat.

Between thirteen, when her periods started, and fourteen she put on three-and-a-half stone and I couldn't pretend any longer that everything was normal. She'd developed terrible acne, problems with her knees and ankles, was having constant headaches and was desperately unhappy at school. She's a bright and conscientious girl, but her size had isolated her. She wasn't able to take part in any activities and while her friends were suddenly talking about boys, she'd become a complete outsider.

Tim and I have always had a pretty good relationship with Christine and one night we all sat down to talk about it. We discussed diets. I was deliberately very up-beat about the success a diet could have (though I can't say I'm a walking advertisement). She was much less certain, saying that she didn't have the will-power to stick to one and anyway she'd become so faddish that there was practically nothing she could eat without feeling ill. And in truth, if you ignored the crisps, cakes and burgers, she'd reached a stage where she more or less lived on cereals and milk. Nothing was resolved and I remember ending that evening feeling pretty hopeless.

It was an article in the local paper that put me on to The NuTron Diet. I was particularly struck that the piece linked overweight to a number of what I'd call sickly symptoms - a good few of which Christine had. She wasn't keen on having her blood sample taken but agreed after I told her it was quite painless these days. Neither of us was prepared for the embarrassment. Christine was so fat the only vein the doctor could find was in her groin. The only saving grace was that it was a lady doctor otherwise, I swear, she'd have run out and thrown herself under the passing traffic.

That wasn't a good start. I can't say I thought things got better when we received the results of her test - because I didn't believe that her main intolerance could be rabbit and trout, which she'd never eaten in her life. There were a few other things there that she didn't eat, either, celery, almonds and turnips. I remember feeling a dull anger because I thought we were being taken for a ride. But I didn't say any of this.

The other main things were salt, potato and tomato - the very stuff of junk food. Christine was also intolerant to the lactose in milk, which didn't surprise me, but not to any of the grains which, by the same token, I did find surprising - as I say, milk and cereals were the staples of her eating and it seemed to me that if she was intolerant to one thing she ate all the time, she should be intolerant to the other. She also showed a candida reaction, which ruled out sugar and chocolate.

I can't say it was easy agreeing a diet that my daughter could stick to, but it was terribly valuable that the safe side of the test pointed her towards things she could have, which gave her confidence, and she was suddenly amenable to eating things she'd liked in the past - sliced turkey, tinned tuna, cottage cheese and pineapple. She developed a liking, too, for brie and Ryvita and for the first time ever began to eat some vegetables. Initially she thought the Lactolite, with which we replaced full milk, disgusting, but by mixing it with a little soya cream I made it at least palatable.

I don't know whether Christine had withdrawal symptoms or not, she wouldn't talk about it and I didn't press the issue, although over the first few days I heard her crying in her room. If she did, it was worth it. At the end of the first week she'd lost six pounds, which we both thought was fairly miraculous. At the end of a month she'd lost two stone. A month later she's dropped another twelve pounds.

I've had to buy Christine a new school uniform and she's so happy I can't believe that just changing what she's eating - because I wouldn't say she's on a diet - can have had such a dramatic effect. What's also wonderful is that her acne has completely disappeared - her skin is beautiful."

* * *

Cindy Driscoll. Age: 28. Height: 5ft. 9in.
Weight before The NuTron Diet: 10st. 6lbs.
Television Presenter.

"Every woman's looks matter to her, but when your job depends on the way you look you have to take action when it's necessary and I do. Television cameras are cruel - they exaggerate what they see. If you're on the thin side they make you look gaunt; if you're a few pounds over, they make you look podgy.

I'm a big girl and well developed through years of tennis and skiing. When I was younger I did a bit of modelling. But I do love my grub, there are times when I binge atrociously - and in this business the opportunities are virtually unavoidable - and I like a drink. I don't mind being six or eight pounds over my ideal weight, but once I slide past that line I take myself off to a health farm. I've tried dieting on my own, but my lifestyle doesn't allow me to stick with anything and I haven't the patience for all that calorie counting.

What fascinated me about The NuTron Diet was that I could see it wasn't a diet at all - just a sensible way of eating and one which, probably, I could live with. If it worked, that is. Frankly, I thought it was probably more a piece of clever marketing than anything else. But when it comes to slimming I'm as eager to be convinced as the next woman.

I had to steel myself to have a blood sample taken. The sight of blood - anyone's - makes me squeamish. A cameraman once fell over in the studio just before we went on air and cut his head and I fainted and had to be replaced. When it came to it, however, it was over before I realised. There I was, eyes firmly squeezed shut, waiting for the needle to plunge in, and the nurse's voice said: "Now, dear, that wasn't so bad, was it?". Haven't things improved!

I honestly don't know what I expected to see in my test results. Part of me rather thought that as I'm so healthy I wouldn't have any intolerances at all. The banned list gave me my comeuppance - nineteen items!

Top of the tree was tannin - and in a business of devoted coffee drinkers, I'm a tea drinker. So move to herbal tea, which like most women I quite like anyway (just as most men loathe it). And no more red wine - okay, I like white, too. And who cares about plums, raisins and currants? But what about baker's yeast, the next on the list? No cakes or biscuits, fine, I'm always giving them up, but no bread? Impossible! But then a little reflection - what's wrong with soda bread? No egg white? Okay again, the cakes and the biscuits into which egg white possibly goes are out already and I can live without eggs, poached, fried, boiled or scrambled. Sesame seed? Well, I've never seen soda bread with sesame seed. Peanuts? The only ones I like are in the strip cartoon. Onions? Yes, I'll miss onions, and I can't think of a substitute for that, and garlic and green pepper. Shrimp and salmon? Ouch. Lettuce? Are you kidding?

I can't remember what the others were. Overall, in total honesty, doing without all the items has been no real hardship. But now that I know more about food intolerance I realise how lucky I am in that my banned list is so easy on me.

THE NUTRON DIET

I started off with a healthy degree of "maybe-ism". Now I'm such a devotee of the diet I try to get almost everyone I meet interested. I lost seven pounds in about twelve days and I didn't even notice!"

EVERYTHING YOU WANT TO KNOW
ABOUT FOOD INTOLERANCE...
and weren't afraid to ask

More than three thousand people have already taken The NuTron Test, discovered the foods to which they're intolerant and removed them from their diet. But almost everyone has had questions. While we've tried to cover everything you need to know earlier in this book, some points are worth emphasising and others worth expanding.

What follows is a compilation of the most common questions people have asked us - and some of the more interesting ones.

- Dr Patrick Kingsley

I understand the explanation of how food intolerance lets undigested food through the intestinal wall into the bloodstream, but I don't understand why the body lets it happen. Surely it should adapt?

Part of the answer is that we used to rotate our foods to a certain extent; we ate seasonally, when foods were available. The paradox is that now most foods are available all the time, and there are so many more of them, we tend constantly to eat the same few things. The result is that we are overloading our systems with these foods and if the body can't cope with some of them, they're likely to cause an intolerant reaction. The less often you eat such a food the less likely you are to develop an intolerance to it. In fact, for some people with definite eating problems, one of the ways of coping is a rotation diet in which foods are put into families according to biological classifications and eaten only once in, say, four days, or seven, according to the rotation devised. It's tedious, but then much less so than the symptoms.

As a piece of general advice, I tell all my patients to ring the changes in what they eat and that advice holds good for anyone who's taken The NuTron Test. It amazes and alarms me that people have so few things on a regular basis - buttered toast and a cup of coffee for breakfast, for instance, day after day. That very narrowness is a potential invitation for food intolerances to build up.

In all honesty, nobody knows why a reaction to any substance occurs or why it's often such a selective sensitivity. Why does an asthmatic who quite clearly reacts to cat hair not react to dog hair? Indeed some people may react to a long-haired cat and not a short-haired cat. Why do some people react to wool and not feathers? We are all exposed to grass pollen every summer of our life and yet one year we may develop hay fever. Whether we ever will have the answer I don't know. Presumably intolerances occur because of some genetic weakness which makes it more likely you will react to something; more to the point, genetic predisposition tends to indicate which particular part of your body is going to react - lungs, joints. We all have a certain level of tolerance to stress, to pain, to anything. Then after a time we can't take it any more. So it is with the accumulation of poisons in our body. There's a build-up - and then something perhaps incidental comes along and breaks the camel's back. If you have a genetic weakness, that's likely to be where the reaction will be produced. Many people have a weight problem which is allied to some other condition.

What's important about The NuTron Diet is that it's not only a means to helping people slim, it's also an application of preventative medicine from which they'll benefit in the longer run. Various studies which have been done on large numbers of people in relationship to the eating or avoidance of foods clearly demonstrate that a certain kind of diet can lead to, or appear to lead to, less disease and greater longevity. It's perfectly reasonable to suggest that, carried out on fit and well people to tell them what foods they are intolerant to and which they should avoid, The NuTron Test will give them a healthier future than they would otherwise have had.

That people have food intolerances sounds logical, but why isn't the subject better known?

It's fair to say that, at present, the subject is on the fringe of medicine and yet there is a plethora of published studies proving the relationship between food reactions and various diseases. Notable is a collection of references by the Department of Medicine at Edinburgh University Western General Hospital entitled 'Food Sensitivities and the Brain', which contains 1,750 articles published in journals regularly read by doctors. While some go back to the last century, over 50% have been published in the last two decades.

There are many reasons why food intolerance hasn't become acceptable to mainstream medicine. Most doctors regard medicine as a science - rather than the art I consider it to be - and a science must be able to prove its claims; if it can't - and where food intolerance is concerned that's basically been the case - then it can be ignored. There's also the fact that modern medicine is often considered to be the study of drugs on biological systems, rather than a way of getting people better. To a very large extent, the pharmaceutical companies lead doctors by the nose. They're wooed by rival drug representatives many times a year, entertained, offered support for studies involving new drugs, given the opportunity to present a resulting paper at some overseas conference. Doctors are trained to think in terms of using drugs - and to be fair, many patients have benefited from them - but the way the companies do their business means that kind of thinking is over-emphasised.

On the other hand, there are many, many doctors who are aware of food intolerance. They simply haven't been able to set about identifying them. The way the National Health Service is run means GPs just don't have the time in most cases to embark on something as difficult and long-winded as an elimination diet - which works despite its drawbacks. What doctors have needed is an acceptable, reliable test which can be applied easily. That's what the NuTron blood test is. I believe it could rapidly change the way medicine is applied and at last give food intolerance its rightful importance.

Is food intolerance a modern phenomenon, or have people always had this problem?

Overweight and conditions such as arthritis have been around for a very long time so, therefore, has food intolerance. Why people today are showing greater signs of suffering from it is because of a combination of reasons: the wide range of foods freely available to us which means we don't rotate our diets; a considerable increase in the total toxic load on our bodies in terms of chemicals in food and the atmosphere and the general levels of pollution; and the increased level of stress induced by modern living. All of this diminishes our tolerance to everything. Any symptom can be caused by anything, but foods play such an important part in our existence that removing those that are causing intolerances is the most obvious way of diminishing a particular toxic load.

Have I been intolerant to the same foods since childhood?

It's very difficult to answer this because nobody has done any studies, which themselves would be difficult. You'd have to test a child, discover its intolerant foods, ensure it did *not* avoid them, and test again in adulthood to check that the intolerances were still present. It's likely you've been intolerant to the same foods since childhood, if you had symptoms in childhood; but it's also possible that you've developed intolerances later on in life.

Once I've been tested and found out what foods I must avoid, do I have to do that for the rest of my life?

Once you've found out what foods you are intolerant to, you must avoid them totally for the first month, and stick whole-heartedly to your list of safe foods. During that month the diet is, in effect, a diagnostic one.

Once you've given your body a chance to recover by avoiding your intolerant foods, your tolerance to them improves and you should be able to eat some of them at least occasionally without the slightest reaction. What's interesting is that when you've avoided a particular food and then re-introduced it, you can easily observe whether you still react to it - or not. And yet when you were eating it regularly you had no idea that you were "suffering" a reaction. What you've done is unmask your symptoms. On the strictest elimination diet which allows only bottled water for five days, an intolerant food re-introduced very soon after that period practically blows a patient apart. If there's a reaction after avoiding an intolerant food for a month, it'll usually be much less severe.

The NuTron Diet encourages you to re-introduce foods after a month, but with great caution. If you like to eat a particular food such as chocolate, you may find that you can have it, say, once a week, without a reaction. Some people, however, find they have to wait longer than a month.

Will The NuTron Diet ensure that I'm getting everything I need, bearing in mind I'm having to cut certain things out, which may mean an unbalanced diet?

Throughout this book we've stressed that avoiding food intolerances is only half of what you must do to eat healthily. The other half is to eat from the list of foods which The NuTron Test has indicated is safe for you - and to eat from it as widely as possible.

But we have no control over the way in which you apply the results of your test. Some people may be too narrowly selective in what they choose to eat from their safe list, in which case there's the possibility they could run the risk of a nutritional deficiency. That's why we suggest that everyone who follows the diet also takes a simple nutritional supplement.

In a book of this sort, we can only give general advice which may not be specific enough for you as an individual. If at any time, you are concerned about your health, you must consult your doctor.

You say everybody is unique - that it's a quirk of fate as to what food they are intolerant to. But doesn't heredity come into it?

We have to say that it does. At present, we don't understand heredity properly, but in the future we will; it is a study that is now getting a great deal of attention. In my own family, my mother used to have migraines -

though she died too long ago for me to know what the cause was - my eldest brother gets migraines if he eats cheese, I get migraines if I eat chocolate, my elder son gets migraines if he eats peanuts. Nobody has done any chromosomal studies, but I think you'd agree that migraines run in my family. Certainly it's heredity. But more to the point, if I don't eat chocolate, I don't get migraines. The heredity mechanism, the predisposition, merely suggests what part of your body is going to react. If you can identify what the triggering factor is, you're able to do something about it. That's precisely what our blood test does for you.

I've got a bit lost trying to understand the part hypoglycaemia and candida play in being overweight. Does everybody who is overweight have hypoglycaemia? Can you lose weight and still suffer from it?

Understanding the part hypoglycaemia (low blood sugar) and candida play in being overweight does require a little lateral thinking.

Hypoglycaemia is an exaggerated response to too much sugar and you don't actually have to have low levels of sugar in your blood to have the symptoms. You can change from a high level of blood sugar to a lower level, but if the rate of fall is fast enough the symptoms can appear. These can be light-headedness, palpitations, sweating, a sense of unreality and feeling really awful. Hunger may or may not be a symptom. Some children can become severely hyperactive, or aggressive, and in extreme cases suffer an epileptic attack. You can equate what happens with coming down in an aeroplane. Your ears are fine when the plane is at 35,000 feet and again when you're on the ground. It's the bit in between that can cause distress - and the quicker a plane descends the greater the problem of equalising the air pressure in your ears can be.

Hypoglycaemia is usually produced by a person having too much sugar over a long period. The body tries to control the situation through its insulin mechanism, which lowers the blood sugar level when it gets too high - and it does this by getting the sugar out of the blood. If sugar stores of glycogen are full, the body converts such sugar into fat and deposits it. Hence the overweight. Over time, the insulin mechanism switches on too acutely, blowing the blood sugar down very rapidly - and thus inducing the hypoglycaemia or the symptoms of it.

Not everyone who's overweight has hypoglycaemia - that is, low blood sugar. Some do, some don't. In the process of losing weight you can still suffer from it. In some people hypoglycaemia can be corrected by taking adequate supplements of chromium.

The candida organism is a yeast, a mould, which exists harmlessly in the intestinal tract, controlled by far greater numbers of friendly bacteria. It's when these friendly bacteria are killed off by antibiotics, or by an attack of gastro-enteritis, or the potentially harmful bacteria are promoted by steroids (both oral and inhaled), by the contraceptive pill, hormone replacement therapy, or by a diet high in refined carbohydrates - that the candida organisms, which are much tougher, can become pathogenic. Sometimes they escape into the bloodstream, where they feed on sugar. When that happens, the blood sugar level falls - and you become hypoglycaemic. This makes you feel you want to eat something sugary which you do, driving up your blood sugar level. The insulin mechanism is triggered to bring it down - and more fat is deposited in your tissues.

You can have candida and not have a particularly sweet tooth. This is when the candida has multiplied but is still confined, at least in the main, to the bowel, where the symptoms are likely to be bloating and gas. Candida alone doesn't automatically make people put on weight, but what it does do is contribute to the leaky gut syndrome caused by food intolerance. Removing the food intolerances cuts down on the bowel's ability to allow both undigested food - and candida - through into the bloodstream.

Once I've eliminated candida - and assuming I stick to my safe food list - will it come back?
Candida is a far, far wider-spread problem than the medical profession acknowledges and that's because, unless it's present in one of its obvious forms, such as thrush in the mouth or vagina, it's difficult to identify.

Candida can cause psychological problems such as depression, anxiety, and lack of concentration; and physical complaints such as nausea, abdominal pain, acne, headache, sinusitis, cystitis, pre-menstrual syndrome, joint pains, fatigue - and many others too numerous to mention but not forgetting hypoglycaemia. Yet a person could have some of these symptoms without candida, or similar types of organisms, being the cause. The NuTron Test's ability to identify the presence of candida could be of major medical significance.

Unfortunately, even if you stick to your safe food list, it's a possibility that you won't entirely get rid of the organism or, if you do, that it will not come back. Once candida has gained a reasonable foothold in the bowel it's not that easy to eradicate it simply by changing your diet. Many people can, if their symptoms aren't severe, by avoiding refined carbohydrates and most foods of a yeast type - baker's and brewer's yeast, cheese, melon, mushroom, all vinegars except pure chemical acetic acid. But those who have severe candidiasis or have suffered from it for a protracted period should take other measures. The most important is to put back into the bowel in large numbers the "good guy" flora that have been killed off in the ways I've described. To achieve this I recommend taking Biodophilus (from Biocare, Tel: 021 433 3727), though there are similar preparations on the market. In some cases nutritional supplements may be needed and an anti-fungal drug such as Nystatin.

Having had a NuTron Test I've discovered I have candida. But in all the years I've been going to the doctor with various complaints he's never once mentioned candidiasis. Obviously it's possible to have it without knowing it?

I'm afraid it is. As we've said earlier, candidiasis isn't picked up by doctors as often as it should be.

Here's a check list to determine the likelihood of your suffering from it:

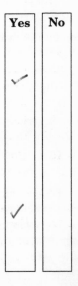

	Yes	No
1 Have you had a lot of antibiotics, either recently or in the past?	✓	
2 Have you suffered fairly frequently from diarrhoea or had gastro-enteritis a few times?		
3 Do you suffer from persistent thrush?		
4 Do you have, or have you suffered from, endometriosis?	✓	
5 Do you suffer from premenstrual tension, or painful or irregular periods?		

		Yes	No
6	Are you on the contraceptive pill, or were you in the past for more than a year?		
7	Are you having hormone replacement therapy, or have you had it in the past for more than a year?	✓	
8	Have you had corticosteroid drugs, such as prednisolone, dexamethasone, betamethasone, by mouth or ACTH injections?		
9	Have you ever had three months or more of inhaled steroids such as Beconase for rhinitis, or Becotide or Bextasol for asthma?		
10	Have you had three or more pregnancies?		
11	Do you have cysts in your breasts?		
12	Do you suffer from diabetes?		
13	Do you suffer from such symptoms as mental confusion, mental fatigue, loss of concentration, forgetfulness, depression or mood swings?	✓	
14	Do you suffer from periodic or regular skin problems such as chronic urticaria (hives), psoriasis or fungal infections such as athletes' foot, or a rash between your buttocks or in your groin?	✓	
15	Do you suffer from abdominal symptoms such as pain, bloating, constipation, diarrhoea, wind or indigestion?		
16	Do you suffer from cystitis, soreness or itching in the vaginal area, vaginitis or loss of interest in sex?	✓	

	Yes	No
17 Do you have headaches, muscle and joint pains or incoordination?	✓	
18 Do you crave sugar, sugary foods such as chocolate or cakes, or yeast foods such as cheese, bread, alcohol or vinegar?	✓	
19 Do you feel generally unwell with a number of vague minor symptoms that no-one can explain?	✓	
20 Do you feel unwell in damp or mouldy conditions such as cellars or caves, or in damp weather?	✓	
21 Do you feel unwell when gardening, especially in winter?	✓	
22 Do you have multiple allergies, and react to chemicals in the environment such as petrol and diesel fumes, North Sea Gas or perfume?		

Questions 1-8

If you've answered yes to one question, it's *possible* you have candidiasis

If you've answered yes to two questions, it's *probable* you have candidiasis

If you've answered yes to three questions, it's *almost definite* you have candidiasis

Questions 9-22

If you've answered yes to three questions, it's *possible* you have candidiasis

If you've answered yes to six questions, it's *probable* you have candidiasis

If you've answered yes to nine questions, it's *almost definite* you have candidiasis

THE NUTRON TEST HAS ALREADY PROVED TO BE A VERY USEFUL WAY OF CONFIRMING CASES.

My test shows that my major intolerance is to crab which, as far as I know, I've never eaten. How can I be intolerant to something I've never had? Surely an intolerance is something that builds up?

What the questioner is saying sounds logical. But most foods consist of a very large number of chemical substances and if you break them down you find there are similarities between surprisingly different types. It's possible that someone develops an intolerance while they are in the womb. But it's much more likely that the chemical substances in some food or foods to which you are intolerant just happen to come together in crab.

I see from the list of foods I must avoid that I don't eat some of them anyway. Yet one or two of these things are higher up the list than some of the things I've been used to eating all the time. That leads me to ask: Is one food intolerance as bad as another?

Theoretically, the food highest on the list - which produces a major reaction on your blood cells - is the one which should be avoided at all costs. But you may not eat it as often as one lower down the list and this second food - which because you eat it more often does more damage to the neutrophils in your blood - can contribute more to your total of symptoms.

It's possible that some of the foods on your positive list aren't clinically very important - certain foods don't produce major reactions, or even any reactions, when they're re-introduced into the diet. But it's better to go over the top and avoid more rather than less for the first

107

four weeks. After that, all the foods can be put back in
on a periodic basis if you so desire. Giving your body a
four-week rest from an intolerant food may well build
up your tolerance to the extent that you can eat it
regularly; but it may be that you can only eat it
occasionally if you aren't to suffer a reaction.

While most people lose their sensitivity to an
intolerant food the longer they avoid it, some people,
definitely a minority, seem to become more sensitive.
However, if they continue to avoid it, say for a number
of months, even their intolerance will gradually
diminish. A very small number of people have to stay off
some foods for ever.

**I have a friend who is really gross and never stops
eating. But never mind the fancy medical words - she's
fat because she's greedy, surely.**

No fat people come out of prisoner of war camps.
Clearly, if you eat practically nothing, you must lose
weight. Conversely, if you eat considerable amounts,
you will put weight on. Established very-low calorie
diets cut people down to less than 800 calories a day and
can go as low as 400 calories and considerable weight
loss can be achieved on them. But it's extremely
difficult, if not impossible, to maintain that level of
intake and the price of following them is constant
feelings of hunger and misery; and when people go back
to nothing more than reasonable eating, they invariably
put the weight back on again.

If a person has food intolerances and eats a lot they
will not only get heavier, they're likely to continue to do
so. Having said that, there are people who, once they
avoid their intolerant foods, can eat what to most of us
are unreasonable amounts and they still lose weight -
though they'd probably lose more if they ate less.

What it demonstrates is that the medical profession and the slimming industry, which both try to pigeon-hole people by saying everybody responds in the same way, are clearly wrong. People have to have their food intolerances identified individually - and that is what The NuTron Test does.

I've always understood that some people are fat because they have trouble with their glands. Food intolerance hasn't got anything to do with their problem has it?

It most certainly has - the right dietary approach will make a big difference, though it may not make as much difference as it can until something's done about the glandular problem. Someone may not lose weight on The NuTron Diet if they have a thyroid deficiency. Again, the medical profession will say that if the thyroid gland is not putting out a normal amount of hormone it will show in a blood test. This is factually correct. But it doesn't take account of the fact that, while the thyroid is producing the required amount of hormone, there can be something wrong with the utilisation of it by the cells. This can be shown by taking temperatures regularly. A normal body temperature is 37^0 C; if someone is consistently 36^0 C and below during the daytime, there's likely to be something wrong with their thyroid mechanism. People may also fail to lose weight if they have a problem with their adrenal glands, which means they have a sluggish metabolism and don't burn up their food intake properly.

I'm afraid it's also true - as we've emphasised earlier - that for some women who are on the Pill or HRT, The NuTron Diet may have limited success. Both can interfere with the weight loss which would otherwise occur, having some kind of blocking effect which at this moment we don't understand. "However, despite these problems a number of people have reported very favourable results. Indeed, in some instances their symptoms have improved so significantly that it has been possible to stop the HRT. Of course, this has only been done with the full co-operation of their physician."

Another mother I see when collecting the children from school has been on a milk-only diet since Easter and she's lost six stone. Doesn't that prove that other diets work, which you say isn't so?

I would never say that other diets can't work. As I've already explained, if you practically don't eat you can emaciate yourself - though, on the other hand, it's quite possible to be just above starvation level on perhaps 500 calories and gain weight. And, let me reiterate, it's virtually impossible to stay on a very low-calorie diet for any length of time.

I accept someone can lose stones on a milk-only diet. The point, however, is that if someone were intolerant to milk they would have difficulty. I'm afraid that once this person comes off her milk-only diet and returns to even a relatively modest intake of 1,500 calories, the weight will accumulate once more.

Such a restricted diet is obviously crashingly boring - and someone on it needs to take extra minerals and vitamins to ensure they remain in good health. The beauty of The NuTron Test is that it doesn't head you off on to a very restricted diet - and it allows you to eat quite normally.

EVERYTHING YOU WANT TO KNOW...

**I can't believe I've been dieting and calorie counting
all these years to absolutely no avail. Indeed,
at different times I have lost weight, though you're
right in thinking I've never managed to keep the extra
poundage off. How could the world believe calorie
counting was the way to slim if it's
just a load of rubbish?**

Calorie counting in itself is not a load of rubbish. All
food consists of calories and self-evidently the number of
calories you take into your body plays a vital part in the
state of your health, of which your weight is a part. But
this is to miss the point. If some of your calories are
coming from foods to which you're intolerant you may
lose weight in the short term, but you're not correcting
your long-term problems. Once you come off a diet the
weight goes back on. If you don't know what your food
intolerances are and don't eliminate them, all you're
doing is "yo-yo" dieting.

**I've always understood that exercise is not only
important to my health, it's an important additional or
alternative way of losing weight. What are your views?**

There have now been enough scientific studies,
supported by a mass of anecdotal evidence, to endorse
the opinion that exercise is a very poor way of helping
people to lose weight, although some recent studies
have suggested it can be helpful. I think it's of very
little value - the necessary work-rate is high relative
to the effective return. And for those with a
significant weight problem, exercise can actually be
harmful. Once a weight loss has been achieved by
diet, however, exercise is beneficial and pleasurable,
not least because it stirs up the metabolism and tones
the muscles.

I've read that almost everybody is intolerant to a handful of things like coffee, tea, eggs and bread. If I excluded these things would I lose weight without bothering to take The NuTron Test?

Perfectly possible - if those things happened to be your particular intolerogenic foods. But if there were others to which you were more intolerant, there would probably be no weight loss or, if there were, it would be considerably less than if your major intolerogens had been identified and avoided.

You've said that an elimination diet, for all the difficulties of applying it, is a good method for finding out a person's food intolerances. In what respect is The NuTron Test different or better?

The elimination diet has stood as the "gold standard", but only because there hasn't been a good blood test. The NuTron Test is a good blood test - and it's a tremendous leap forward on the elimination diet.

The elimination diet proceeds by guesswork. The principle is that if you remove a food from someone's diet and they feel better, you then re-introduce it and they feel worse, you have acceptable evidence that they're intolerant to that food. In practice, patients start either by fasting totally, or by cutting their intake to perhaps three or four hopefully safe foods, for five to seven days, after which the orderly re-introduction of items begins, one by one.

The difficulties, however, are after what period do you re-introduce a food to a diet, how much of it do you re-introduce, how frequently do you re-introduce other foods, and when a reaction does take place what precisely is it in relation to? If you've re-introduced three different foods in a day and you feel ill the next day, which of those foods is responsible for the symptoms? You can very easily come up with the wrong answer.

Another serious problem involves what symptoms a person suffers as a result of an intolerance to a particular food. If re-introducing a food means a headache, even a migraine, the person may think it worth it, even if it has to happen twenty or thirty times over the two or three months it can take to identify all their intolerances. But what if a symptom is potentially dangerous, such as an asthmatic or epileptic attack?

The NuTron Test helps to identify the foods to which someone is intolerant with a high degree of certainty. The safe list gives them an average of around eighty foods that is wide enough for them not to bother with re-introducing intolerant items unless they specifically want to. Even if they do, the purpose isn't to see whether they react, as in the elimination diet, but, rather, to see that they *don't*.

**I know The NuTron Diet works because I've already
lost over two stone, but I simply can't understand how
I'm able to eat as much as I like of my safe foods.
Explain this to me: presumably my body can
only take out so much goodness from what I eat - why
doesn't the rest get turned into fat?**

Some studies have been done which show that basic levels of energy or use of oxygen increase when people are on a low-calorie diet - though when you go down into the 400-500 calorie range your metabolism actually slows down. Until now, however, because of the difficulties of applying an elimination diet - and because of the widespread resistance of the medical profession to the very idea of food intolerance - relatively few people have been tested. That means very few if any studies have been done in this area. The only way I can answer this question at present is by saying that removing your food intolerances must in some way stimulate your metabolism, which makes you burn up your food intake more quickly and efficiently. Perhaps food intolerance suppresses thyroid function or simply acts as a dampener on the metabolism.

A study of the relationship between food intolerance and metabolism would be of enormous medical benefit and I hope than now The NuTron Test makes it possible, the idea will be taken up.

You say most really excessive overweight is retained fluid. But are you saying someone who is, say, six or seven pounds overweight, is also retaining fluid?

I don't automatically say most excessive overweight is retained fluid, but a large proportion of it certainly is. You have only to look at what happens to women in the pre-menstrual phase when half a stone can go on in a few days. There's no way that can be deposited fat. When you consider that such women often feel bloated at other times, it seems reasonable to assume that, in the very overweight, at least twice that amount of weight is retained fluid. Much of this is locked between the fat cells. As the fat cells diminish in size, they release more fluid, too.

It would be a mistake to think that a person who has perhaps only ten pounds to lose is suffering entirely from deposited fat. We have yet to compile statistical evidence, but I'd say that about half of this amount is retained fluid.

I've had no luck with diets, though God knows I've tried enough. Now I don't bother. I feel very depressed about the way I look and truthfully I eat to try to relieve the depression. If I'm tested and find out what I shouldn't have, will the depression go away?

The depression caused directly by your food intolerances

should go away. Then when you realise that The NuTron Diet is helping you lose weight, you'll be so encouraged by your weight loss that the depression which is caused by the way you look should also lift. It's fair to say that some people's depression is caused by a lack of nutrients; for them it may take a little longer, while the body replenishes itself, though they may have to supplement it with vitamins and minerals.

For years I've suffered from such bad cellulite I don't dare get into a bathing costume. I'd like to lose weight - but if you can convince me I'll definitely lose my cellulite I'll be off for a blood test before you can say Jane Fonda!

Cellulite will begin to go once the foods that are causing your problems are eliminated. What will happen is that the permeability of the intestine will be reduced, thereby cutting down on the amount of fat you absorb from a given meal. You can, of course, help the process by reducing your fat intake.

The safe diet on its own should ensure that many people's cellulite will go without them taking other measures. Where it's a particular problem, however, things can be speeded up by some gentle exercise - walking to the shops instead of taking the car is a good beginning, as are some sit-ups. Remember, the cellulite isn't just stretching the skin, it's in all the tissues surrounding muscles, so it's made them lax. Some exercise to tone them up makes sense.

I've put on a lot of weight during pregnancy which I'm sure is unhealthy. I understand what The NuTron Diet does in rough terms, but I don't know whether it's sensible to be tested now or after I've had the baby.

I would prefer any woman to eliminate her food

intolerances from her diet before she gets pregnant, but it's perfectly safe, and sensible, to go on the diet at any stage during pregnancy, the earlier the better. The diet will help a woman ensure she doesn't put on enormous amounts of weight (it's a fact that women who have a tendency to being overweight during pregnancy also tend to become excessively heavy when they take the Pill or HRT). The other value of the diet is that it'll help ensure a mother doesn't pass on potential problems to the child in her womb.

I always recommend that a woman takes a supplement of vitamins and minerals during pregnancy and also while she's breast feeding. It's important that a woman should seek professional advice at the right time.

I've suffered several miscarriages and there's been no real explanation. Would eliminating my food intolerances give me a better chance of carrying a baby to full term?

I had a patient who reached the stage of thirty-two weeks pregnant when she became extremely toxic. She was admitted to hospital, where she was told the baby was dying and only complete rest was likely to save it. She discharged herself, came straight to see me, I identified her problems as best I could (this was before The NuTron Test was available) and took her off certain foods. She'd started to suffer severe headaches and felt extremely ill, but by the evening she saw me her symptoms had started to disappear and soon the baby was kicking again. When subsequently her son was born, there was clear evidence of separation of the placenta from the womb about the time she'd gone into hospital. I relate this particular story because it's stayed in my mind - the mother named her child after me. But

I've dealt with other women who've had multiple miscarriages and then produced the most superb baby after having their food intolerances identified. Food intolerances are not the only cause of miscarriage and I would recommend that anyone who's already suffered a miscarriage and still wants a baby or who's worried that she might have a miscarriage, should contact Foresight, 28, The Paddock, Godalming, Surrey GU7 1XD (Tel: 0483 427839), enclosing a s.a.e.

Generally speaking, any woman who eliminates her food intolerances - and takes the precaution of having additional nutrient supplements - will significantly increase her chances of avoiding difficulties during pregnancy. It will help her control her weight and make her pregnancy altogether more pleasant - it will significantly reduce, if not abolish, morning sickness. I recommend that an expectant mother taking The NuTron Test discusses the outcome with a dietician or nutritionist.

Most women have cravings of the jam-on-kippers type during pregnancy. Has food intolerance anything to do with this?

An intriguing question and fascinating to speculate - but I don't know the answer. Some cravings can certainly be caused by specific nutritional deficiencies of chromium, zinc and/or magnesium, and vitamin B6. It may well be because of these deficiencies that the appetite system and the brain are affected in some way that might compare with what happens in anorexia and bulimia. When enough pregnant or about-to-be-pregnant women have taken The NuTron Test, it'll be interesting to amass some evidence.

During my labour I drank a lot of tea which I've now found out I can't have due to my intolerance to tannin. In the last half hour before delivery, my baby went into sudden and unexplained "foetal distress". Could this have been the tea reaching her in a massive dose?

A distinct possibility. Tannin is a very nasty irritant for adults, never mind a baby at the foetal stage.

Just after I gave birth to my daughter I had an injection of ergotamine to contract the womb. Since this is usually made from rye and I have since tested intolerant to gluten, would you say this was probably the cause of the 'baby blues' I suffered?

I don't think Ergotamine could cause a problem in relation to food intolerance. When it was manufactured from rye it came from the non-gluten portion; nowadays it's probably chemically produced.

A cause of the "baby blues" could have been your gluten reaction, especially at a time when the hormones had changed significantly, but that was very likely compounded by nutritional deficiencies which are depressingly common in pregnant and breast-feeding women.

Smoking suppresses cravings and therefore when people give up smoking they usually gain weight. This may seem like a silly question - but can smoking suppress food intolerances?

Smoking probably does suppress the desire to eat in some way; more to the point, it blunts the taste perception - smokers don't enjoy food as much as non-smokers. There are plenty of studies which show that when people give up smoking they eat more and that's why they put on weight. Smokers are used to having something in their mouth, so when they give up, many take sweets or chocolate for oral satisfaction purposes.

Some people satisfy that urge by sucking a pebble - which has no fattening dangers!

As to whether smoking suppresses food intolerances, again, I don't know. Very likely it does mask them.

I work outdoors and over the last few years I've had aches and pains in all my joints, for which I was advised to take cod liver oil capsules. My test has now shown that I'm intolerant to cod. Have I been making myself worse by taking these capsules?

Probably not - what we've tested is the fish meat; it's likely that the liver oil has a different intolerogenic potential, although we can't be sure. However, to be safe, it would be sensible to change to another fish oil.

My test showed I was intolerant to gluten, whey, malt and baker's yeast, among other things, which means I've had to give up every kind of bread there is. I can't complain, I've lost twenty-five pounds in two months and I haven't felt so good in years. But I do miss my bread. Any suggestions welcome!

In the days when I used to go round giving talks to self-help groups and the general public I was frequently asked: When you put a person on a tea and coffee-free diet, what do you recommend they drink? I used to reply: "What you're asking me is what can I drink that tastes like tea and coffee but isn't tea or coffee. I'm afraid there isn't anything." The same holds good for bread.

If you're going to be successful on The NuTron Diet, you have to have a positive attitude. Your safe list gives you a very wide choice of things to eat and drink - tell yourself you don't need the others. And be pleased with the way you now look and feel. If you really think you can't live without bread, try a slice. If it makes you feel sick, that's a very good reason for going on avoiding it. You may find the taste disappointing - many people do experience that after abstaining from a favourite food for an extended period. If, however, you find you enjoy it and don't suffer a reaction., fine - though I'd advise you not to overdo it.

Barley is on my list of foods I've got to avoid. I'm partial to a glass of whisky - but how much barley is left in whisky after it's distilled?

The way to discover whether or not something causes you a problem is to try it after the initial four weeks of avoidance. Answering the question more broadly: at the moment we don't know what percentage of ingredients used in the manufacture of different alcoholic drinks is left after the process is completed - it's something we want to investigate in the future. The amount of malt and yeast which remains in British beers and lagers is probably quite high; and the yeast in wine may be significant, at least for some people.

It seems ever so difficult to avoid certain things like whey and corn starch in processed food and I'm sure that applies to other ingredients. Have you any basic advice to offer?

I'm uncompromising on this one. Avoid all packets. It's alarming what an incredible range of foods and chemicals are present in most of them - have you ever wondered why chemicals extend the food shelf-life? If you're trying to avoid your food intolerances, packets simply aren't worth the trouble and risk, besides being of limited nutritional value. My advice on food preparation is: do it the way granny did, before so many things were so readily available on the shelves.

AFTERWORD
Off the back-burner

The NuTron Diet was launched in the autumn of 1993, since when things have moved at startling speed. Countries across Europe have begun to negotiate rights to The NuTron Test - which is expected to launch in the USA in the summer of this year. A number of highly respected nutritional scientists have looked at our findings, endorsed them and, in several cases, have joined us in a variety of research projects. Newspapers and television companies have beaten a path to our door. And the first print run of 'The NuTron Diet' book, published in April, sold out in two weeks.

It would be too sweeping a claim to say that the entire medical profession has woken up to the significance of food intolerance; the degree of ignorance or scepticism that exists about the subject is too great to be broken down overnight. But the list of GPs now sending their patients' blood to us for analysis has risen to the thousands and is growing daily - many doctors are learning about food intolerance because their patients have come to us in the first place. More and more hospitals are contacting us about using The NuTron Test in the furtherance of their work. And our register of clients has swelled to the point where we can barely keep pace with bookings - over 8,000 NuTron Tests have been booked since the beginning of the year and the figure is rising rapidly. All the signs are that, at last, food intolerance has come off the medical back-burner where for so long it has barely simmered because of the lack of a credible test.

Some of the research partnerships we've formed include one with a leading children's hospital to investigate the effects of food intolerance on lactating mothers; infantile asthma, infantile eczema and colic will come under the hospital's future scrutiny. Another is with the University of California in Los Angeles for a major study of eczema; and a third with an ad hoc group, one of whose members is a former Chief Constable, which will conduct some pioneering research into the likelihood that food intolerance plays a part in the behaviour of juvenile offenders. Other partnerships to investigate glue ear, dyslexia and hyperactivity are under discussion or in early stages of development.

At a recent conference, the consultant physician at Stobhill Hospital, Glasgow, Dr Matthew Dunnigan, an expert on fluid retention syndrome, reported that his research has led him to conclude that more than one women in four suffers from fluid retention to some degree. This is in line with our own findings, which we've outlined for you. Contrary to popular belief, perhaps half the weight most people need to lose is fluid, NOT fat, and removing fluid is easy - once you know what causes it.

When we launched The NuTron Diet, we thought that, probably, more people would come to us to achieve weight loss than to seek relief for inflammatory conditions. In fact, there have been almost as many bookings in the second category as in the first. And feedback has shown that even those who've sought our help for a weight problem have also reaped other benefits.

Clare, our 'guinea-pig' for this book, happened to mention recently that she'd had a flaky scalp since her teens and this, she'd suddenly noticed, has cleared up - she hadn't thought to mention the condition during the time we were following her progress.

There are some thirty illnesses of an inflammatory nature. The medical profession, generally, treats these as separate entities. But The NuTron Test clearly indicates that, like overweight, they are multiple symptoms of a single cause - food intolerance.

As long ago as 1982-83, 'The Lancet' published a series of papers on rheumatoid arthritis - which affects one million people in the UK - and on irritable bowel syndrome. These showed that when foods to which individuals are intolerant were removed from their diet, their symptoms disappeared. The success rate was 30% in cases of rheumatoid arthritis and 70% in cases of IBS. Similar published papers have demonstrated improvements in virtually all other inflammatory conditions.

Yet, despite this fairly dramatic evidence, the vast majority of doctors at both GP and consultant level have continued to address their patients' problems in the same old ways, with steroids and anti-inflammatories - that is, treating the symptoms and not the cause. Earlier, we went to some lengths to explain the reasons why this was, the principle one being that overworked GPs, particularly, don't have the time or the experience to run elimination diet procedures. But as we've carried on our research and continued to sift the wealth of published evidence about food intolerance, we've come to realise that there's been a possibly even more significant factor. *None of the research papers on food intolerance explained why the removal of intolerogenic foods should produce the improvements they do.*

Those who were investigating the role food intolerance plays in the inflammatory conditions of arthritis, IBS, asthma, cystitis, eczema, pre-menstrual tension, migraine and the rest (which together affect half the population) hadn't appreciated the part played by neutrophils - the group of white blood cells that food intolerance causes to break down and spill poisonous chemicals into the bloodstream. On the other hand, those researchers who knew that damaged neutrophils were involved in inflammatory illnesses seemed unaware that food intolerance was what caused the cell-group to break down.

Our development of The NuTron Test has enabled us to see the link between the parallel areas of work. Put together, they provide overwhelming evidence that the conclusions about food intolerance we'd independently arrived at were right.

THE SUBJECT OF FOOD INTOLERANCE WAS LIKE AN ENORMOUS JIGSAW THAT NEEDED ONE FINAL PIECE TO COMPLETE THE PICTURE. THAT PIECE WAS THE NUTRON TEST. AS THE PICTURE IS SEEN WITH EVER-INCREASING CLARITY, THERE'S NO DOUBT IN OUR MINDS THAT THE TEST WILL PROVE TO BE ONE OF THE MAJOR MEDICAL MILESTONES OF MODERN TIMES.

If we can change the mind-set of the medical profession generally, with particular reference to those illnesses known to be associated with overweight, there could be an immediate saving on the National Health Service drugs bill of 15%.

Can The NuTron Test really be so simple? Discover from a small blood sample the foods to which you are intolerant, eliminate them from your diet, eat as much as you like of the foods The NuTron Test shows are safe for you - and you should lose weight, or find an improvement in your health, or both?

Yes. We monitored hundreds of people before we put The NuTron Diet on the market. We've monitored thousands since. And the story remains consistent. Many, many clients with inflammatory conditions improve in a way conventional medicine fails to achieve; while of those seeking weight loss, 70% lose half a stone or more in the first four weeks, with 10% losing $1^{1}/2$-2 stone in the first eight weeks.

The Individual Diet Company is a business; it's gratifying to everyone involved that we're flourishing so remarkably. But it's even more gratifying that, in conducting the business, we've already brought relief to so many people suffering pain and misery. One client, confined to a wheelchair for nine years by rheumatoid arthritis, is now walking around her home and garden after a few months on her NuTron Diet - during which, incidentally, she's also lost over three stone. She calls what's happened to her is a miracle. 'It seems unbelievable,' she told us, 'that giving up a few everyday foods has made such a difference.'

Doesn't that say everything?

Patrick Kingsley
Ian Stoakes
May 1994

Angela Holroyd
Thus Fri.

Hornly .

APPENDIX

Anorexia And Bulimia

'The NuTron Diet' is written for people who want to lose weight and who understand that the way to do it is by avoiding the foods to which they're intolerant. It seems important, however, to include something about the slimming nightmares of anorexia and bulimia - conditions that almost certainly are triggered in the first place by a period of harmful dieting.

Sufferers of anorexia nervosa and bulimia nervosa have much in common: an obsessive desire to be thin, accompanied by an over-estimate of their real size and an unrealistic idea of how small their ideal size should be. While both conditions also share such feelings as guilt, worthlessness and hopelessness - and often make their sufferers socially withdrawn - they differ in one major respect.

Anorexics starve themselves to emaciation. Bulimics, who also can go for days or even weeks without eating, then gorge themselves, usually on bulk foods high in calories - before making themselves sick. Bulimics look perfectly normal, but can be overweight. They may purge themselves as many as ten times a day. The majority do so by putting their fingers down their throat to induce the gag reflex. Many take laxatives, diuretics or appetite suppressants. Some drink such things as salt water, washing-up liquid or shampoo.

Both anorexia and its near relative surfaced as a major problem in the late 1970s. Anorexia affects about one girl in a hundred, most of them teenagers - about a quarter of a million in the USA, ten thousand in the UK. An estimated one-third of anorexics develop bulimia, in a slightly older age group.

*All of them have been made
ill by a zinc deficiency.*

There are more than a dozen
or so trace elements, which
are as important to the
human body as vitamins. Of
them, iron and zinc are
needed in the largest amounts
- in the case of zinc, fifteen mg
a day, the equivalent of about
two pinheads a day.

Zinc is needed for just about
everything - it's essential to
over a hundred enzyme
functions, physical and
mental growth, digestion,
keeping the immune system
in working order, wound
healing. It also plays a role in
the way the body handles
carbohydrates and fat.

Zinc is found in both
animal and vegetable protein,
with the highest
concentrations in lean meat,
pig's liver, shellfish and
wheatgerm. However, due
principally to the use of
phosphates in agriculture
and to modern food
processing methods, all trace
elements - which, as their
name suggests, are present
only in minute amounts -
have been much reduced or
even eradicated in most food
stuffs. The majority of
modern diets are now
seriously zinc deficient.
Government figures suggest
that people now get no more

than eight-thirteen mg daily.

Most people cope. But some,
invariably pubescent girls
whose bodies and minds are
undergoing hormonal change -
and who are almost certainly
dieting, thereby reducing
their already deficient zinc
intake - do not.

Usually, the body makes a
sensible distribution of what
it does receive to its various
necessities, rather in the way
a company keeps a number of
projects running even when it
doesn't quite have the cash to
fund them all properly.
Anorexia develops when,
having hit a "cash flow" crisis,
the body decides to shut down
a "project" - in this case, the
utilisation of zinc in the brain.
In addition, instead of using
it, the body passes it out -
with a critical effect on the
normal brain function.
Interestingly enough, it does
the same in hyperactive
children, with a different but
equally disastrous result.

Conventional treatment of
anorexia and bulimia still
includes the use of anti-
depressant drugs,
psychotherapy, and "stepped"
diets that are supposed to
return a sufferer to normal
eating. Yet it's seven years
since Professor Derek Bryce-
Smith, Professor of Organic
Chemistry at Reading

130

University, published his pioneering work, 'The Zinc Solution', which not only showed that such methods are largely a waste of effort, but that the answer is a few pennyworth of zinc - which can begin to have beneficial results within hours.

Sadly, while the average GP will happily prescribe iron tablets for a woman with anaemia, he'd never think that another patient who shows the signs of anorexia needed a similar supplement - which he could ascertain by asking her to taste a teaspoon of zinc solution. What to healthy tastebuds is strong and unpleasant is tasteless to the anorexic. The doctor might also examine the patient's nails: brittle nails with white spots or white horizontal lines are classic signs of zinc deficiency.

What induces the body to reject that which is essential to it isn't yet understood, but tests have shown that where anorexics and bulimics have had foods to which they are intolerant removed from their diets, the absorption mechanism gets switched back on.

Anyone eliminating their food intolerances is highly unlikely to develop anorexia nervosa.

THE NUTRON DIET

As we've emphasised throughout this book, a relationship between food intolerance and a range of chronic medical disorders is clearly indicated in medical literature. Substantial work has been undertaken, for example, into:

Adult on-set diabetes
Anorexia
Arthritis
Asthma
Bronchitis
Bulimia
Crohn's disease
Depression
Eczema
Epilepsy
Irritable bowel syndrome
Migraine

Other conditions linked to food intolerance include:

Acne
Anxiety
Cystitis
Glue ear (otitis media)
Hay fever
Hypertension
Hyperactivity
Multiple sclerosis
Pre-menstrual tension
Post-natal depression
Schizophrenia
Sinusitis
Tonsillitis

Anyone suffering from any of these conditions is likely to benefit from identifying the foods to which they are intolerant and removing them from their diet. If these conditions are allied to a problem of overweight, removing intolerant foods - and sticking to the list of safe foods identified on an individual basis by The NuTron Test - should produce a double benefit.

To provide you with your individual
NuTron Diet
either complete the form
or ring:
0483 203555

132

Discover more about our forthcoming books through Penguin's FREE newspaper...

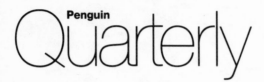

Penguin Quarterly

It's packed with:

- exciting features
- author interviews
- previews & reviews
- books from your favourite films & TV series
- exclusive competitions & much, much more...

Write off for your free copy today to:
Dept JC
Penguin Books Ltd
FREEPOST
West Drayton
Middlesex
UB7 0BR
NO STAMP REQUIRED

READ MORE IN PENGUIN

In every corner of the world, on every subject under the sun, Penguin represents quality and variety – the very best in publishing today.

For complete information about books available from Penguin – including Puffins, Penguin Classics and Arkana – and how to order them, write to us at the appropriate address below. Please note that for copyright reasons the selection of books varies from country to country.

In the United Kingdom: Please write to *Dept. JC, Penguin Books Ltd, FREEPOST, West Drayton, Middlesex UB7 0BR*

If you have any difficulty in obtaining a title, please send your order with the correct money, plus ten per cent for postage and packaging, to *PO Box No. 11, West Drayton, Middlesex UB7 0BR*

In the United States: Please write to *Penguin USA Inc., 375 Hudson Street, New York, NY 10014*

In Canada: Please write to *Penguin Books Canada Ltd, 10 Alcorn Avenue, Suite 300, Toronto, Ontario M4V 3B2*

In Australia: Please write to *Penguin Books Australia Ltd, 487 Maroondah Highway, Ringwood, Victoria 3134*

In New Zealand: Please write to *Penguin Books (NZ) Ltd,182–190 Wairau Road, Private Bag, Takapuna, Auckland 9*

In India: Please write to *Penguin Books India Pvt Ltd, 706 Eros Apartments, 56 Nehru Place, New Delhi 110 019*

In the Netherlands: Please write to *Penguin Books Netherlands B.V., Keizersgracht 231 NL–1016 DV Amsterdam*

In Germany: Please write to *Penguin Books Deutschland GmbH, Friedrichstrasse 10–12, W–6000 Frankfurt/Main 1*

In Spain: Please write to *Penguin Books S. A., C. San Bernardo 117–6º E–28015 Madrid*

In Italy: Please write to *Penguin Italia s.r.l., Via Felice Casati 20, I–20124 Milano*

In France: Please write to *Penguin France S. A., 17 rue Lejeune, F–31000 Toulouse*

In Japan: Please write to *Penguin Books Japan, Ishikiribashi Building, 2–5–4, Suido, Bunkyo-ku, Tokyo 112*

In Greece: Please write to *Penguin Hellas Ltd, Dimocritou 3, GR–106 71 Athens*

In South Africa: Please write to *Longman Penguin Southern Africa (Pty) Ltd, Private Bag X08, Bertsham 2013*

READ MORE IN PENGUIN

A SELECTION OF HEALTH BOOKS

Twins, Triplets and More   Elizabeth Bryan

This enlightening study of the multiple birth phenomenon covers all aspects of the subject from conception and birth to old age and death. It also offers much comfort and support as well as carefully researched information gained from meeting several thousands of children and their families.

Meditation for Everybody   Louis Proto

Meditation is liberation from stress, anxiety and depression. This lucid and readable book by the author of *Self-Healing* describes a variety of meditative practices. From simple breathing exercises to more advanced techniques, there is something here to suit everybody's needs.

Endometriosis   Suzie Hayman

Endometriosis is currently surrounded by many damaging myths. Suzie Hayman's pioneering book will set the record straight and provide both sufferers and their doctors with the information necessary for an improved understanding of this frequently puzzling condition.

My Child Won't Eat   Nick Yapp

Written by a qualified nutritionist, this reassuring guide will provide parents with the facts, help and comfort that will put their minds at rest and allow them to feed their children with confidence.

Not On Your Own   Sally Burningham
The MIND Guide to Mental Health

Cutting through the jargon and confusion surrounding the subject of mental health to provide clear explanations and useful information, *Not On Your Own* will enable those with problems – as well as their friends and relatives – to make the best use of available help or find their own ways to cope.